Why am I where I am, and not in another part of the world?
Why am I who I am, and not a person of another race or belief?
Why am I what I am, instead of being of another occupation or social status?
Because God appointed me to this time, this place, this work, this name.
He gave me this body and this personality, this work to do and these things to do it with because he chose them as best for me.
If the choosing had been mine, I would always wonder if it had been right.
Since God chose, all I need do is to put it to work.

From "A Blade of Grass" by Gladys & Gordon DePree
Page 98, Zondervan Press 1971

Oh Lord, I cannot let you go.
I know you are the one who opens eyes,
whose hands hold healing.
And if the price for that
Is taking to the road without a map,
I will take the road.
And one day,
looking back along the way I have travelled, I will realize there was a plan
That marked the road
You walked with me.

From "Encounters" by Eddie Askew
page 55, Leprosy Mission International, UK, 2004

Doctor Number 49

Grace Warren

of The Leprosy Mission

To Mary Buxey with best wishes – the story of Gods goodness & guidance through a long life of service to Him

Grace Warren July 07

Doctor Number 49

Grace Warren

of The Leprosy Mission

An Autobiography
by Grace Warren with Lesley Hicks

SPCK
AUSTRALIA

Cataloguing in publication data

Warren, Grace.
Doctor number 49: Grace Warren of the Leprosy Mission: an autobiography/with Lesley Hicks.

ISBN 978 1 876106 14 0
ISBN 1 876106 14 X

1. Warren, Grace.
2. Missionaries, Medical — Biography.
3. Surgeons — Australia — Biography.
3. Leprosy — Treatment.
4. Christian life.
I. Hicks, Lesley, 1935-
II. Society for Promoting Christian Knowledge (Australia)

266.0092

Published 2006 by
SPCKA-Australia Publishing
Box 190 Rundle Mall Post Office,
Adelaide, South Australia 5000
Email: publishing@spcka.org.au
www.spcka.org.au

Design – Cogdell Design & Fine Art www.graemecogdell.com.au
Printed by Hyde Park Press

Preface

"So Grace is writing her memoirs. And I've been asked to contribute a few words to the undertaking, part of the reason being that during her time with The Leprosy Mission she called me boss. Her words, not mine. That's the one thing Grace never needed. No need for stimulus or oversight, Grace is and always has been self-motivated - or should that read Spirit-motivated? Her life and work have been one, and her compassionate and very professional care for the sick and underprivileged have been her lifetime's achievement. Guided, not by me, but by the depth and practical outworking of her deep Christian faith.

She has always been ready to share both her faith and her surgical experience with all who would listen. I remember travelling with her once during peak hour on London's Underground, on one of her visits. I'd invited her home for supper. Grace's voice is not the quietest of voices, and her sharing of her recent surgical experiences with me over the 25 minute journey had most of the train carriage fascinated.

She shared her knowledge willingly, travelling widely throughout Asia and further afield. The uniqueness of her knowledge, understanding and prodigious energy brought hope and new life to many, both directly as she treated the individual, and through her teaching of medical personnel at all levels, from paramedical worker to consultant.

Grace is a phenomenon. A totally committed Christian doctor ready and able to take on the world and leave it a better place. It has been a privilege to know her, to share the same ideals, and to be challenged and stimulated by her.

Eddie Askew O.B.E.

Retired International Director
The Leprosy Mission.

Acknowledgements

How can I begin to acknowledge the love, support and prayers given by so many hundreds of people over a lifetime

- To my family and friends who are all very special to me
- To my mentors who have urged me on when the going has been hard
- To my patients in every country who have blessed me as I have ministered to them. In most cases I have not used your true names
- To colleagues who have shown me the importance of a surgeon's precision and detailed work
- To the vast family of The Leprosy Mission who have aided and supported me in my endeavours to expand the work
- To be able to live in a modern age of technology and medication and yet be practical and adaptable and to utilize simple things
- To Lesley Hicks who knows the gift of words and helped me streamline this writing, and to her husband John for many hours spent on the electronic media assisting the project
- To somebody who once said; "It is fun making other people famous"
- To SPCK-Australia for taking me on in the risky business of publishing
- To the many others who helped me greatly, some of whose names appear in the text
- To God my Saviour whom I have known for a life time and who gifted me for this very special ministry –

THANK YOU

Foreword by Professor Bruce Conolly

Dr Grace Warren, AM, MD, MS, FRACS, FRCS, DTM & H

You have in your hands the autobiography of a remarkable humanitarian, Christian medical missionary, pioneer surgeon, teacher and author, Dr Grace Warren.

My close association and friendship with Dr Warren began in 1979 when, with my wife Dr Joyce Conolly, I had the opportunity of visiting the McKean Institute in Chang Mai, Thailand and worked there with her. I was privileged to see her work at first hand and was impressed by the thoroughness of how she examined her patients, making those patients, along with the physiotherapists, understand their respective roles in not only the post-operative management but also the actual surgical procedure. I have studied, taught and practised surgery of the hand and upper extremity in over 20 countries but have never worked with a surgeon who could match Dr Grace in the logic and precision of her surgical technique.

Since then, I have worked with her in Cambodia and in Australia where she is a Consultant Hand Surgeon at the Hand Units of St Luke's and Sydney Hospitals.

From the time she graduated in Medicine from the University of Sydney in January 1954, Dr Grace has devoted her life to the care of her fellow man, especially those with leprosy and related neuropathic conditions. Her experience in this field has been detailed in her book *The Care of Neuropathic Limbs* published in 1999. In this book she has illustrated the principles which can be applied both in sophisticated centres and in the underdeveloped places of the world where there are no resources. She has been a real pioneer in this respect.

In the male dominated world of surgery in Australia in the 1950s, opportunities for women to learn reconstructive surgery were few.

But by the end of the 1960s Dr Warren was running training programs for leprosy surgery in Asia.

Having started her medical career almost unrecognized and as one of the few lady surgeons of her time, she has since then been honoured in many ways – most of which are recorded in the text. The Royal Australasian College of Surgeons recognised her expertise by requesting her to give the Edward Dunlop oration in 2004, and most recently in 2006, she received the Star of Pakistan (Sitari-I-Pakistan – the 3rd highest award Pakistan gives to civilians for humanitarian service to their country). This award recognizes her ongoing work in biannual visits to Pakistan over the past 40 years. This great honour, granted by a Muslim country to a Christian woman for work done in the name of God was, to Dr Warren, the ultimate in pleasure and achievement.

Prior to writing this autobiography, Dr Warren had written 53 scientific papers. This is no mean feat for someone who was told she would have great difficulty in passing the NSW Department of Education Leaving Certificate in 1944!

This autobiography describes her background and experiences in many areas including the Middle East, Africa and Asia, as well as in Western countries.

Dr Warren's principle has been one of regular follow-up. She would spend three weeks or so in a place, returning three months later to assess not only the patients on whom she operated, but also the work of those therapists and doctors whom she had taught and on whom she relied to carry on her work until her return.

In 1959, she accepted a temporary position at the Hong Kong Leprosy Hospital. (This became permanent, and she the superintendent). In 1975, when virtually all the leprosy patients had been treated successfully, that hospital closed. Grace moved her base to the Manorom Hospital in central Thailand and embarked on an enlarged program. From 1975-1989 she conducted in-service training programs in about 10 Asian countries, teaching surgery and therapy techniques. Dr Warren's original contract with The Leprosy Mission was that she would retire when she was 60 years old. Who could imagine this woman of limitless energy and experience ceasing work! Thus her official position as adviser for leprosy and reconstructive surgery for The Leprosy Mission in Asia became renamed "previous adviser".

She continued her missions in Asia, Israel, UK and Africa, but then made more time for her Australian work, providing a consultative and advisory service for the care of patients with neuropathic limbs (feet and hands) and also faces: patients with problems similar to those with leprosy. She has had regular input into more than fifteen public and private hospitals in Sydney, Melbourne and elsewhere in Australia.

There are many adjectives to describe Dr Grace - energetic, resourceful, hardworking, caring, logical, practical, leading by example, strong though never aggressive or judgmental, and all with a sense of humour. The Sydney University year book of 1954 in the annotation for Grace, has quoted from Thackeray, "A good laugh is sunshine in the house" and mentions her skills in the handicrafts of sewing and knitting. Grace can be described as a true lady, in every sense of the word, refined and gentle.

Her life's work, as shown in this autobiography, has improved the lives of thousands of patients with neuropathic limbs so that they can now enjoy with pride and in safety an active and rewarding life.

W Bruce Conolly AM FRCS FRACS FACS

Assoc Professor University of Sydney & University of NSW
Director Overseas Hand Surgery Projects,
St Luke's & Sydney Hospitals

Contents

1

Doctor Number 49

There was the usual long line of patients at the Monday morning Fracture Clinic at Westmead Hospital, Sydney. We had already seen a number of people with chronic foot problems.

That morning in January 2000, after I had seen several diabetic patients, in rolled Daren, a stocky young man in his early thirties. He did not have diabetes but walked with the typical rolling gait of someone who has a problem in keeping his balance – a "sailor's gait", the roll of a drunken sailor – with feet well apart to prevent falling over.

He grinned at me and said, "Well, you're doctor number 49! Can you fix my foot?"

The case notes that I had been given did not help much, so I sat down to listen to his story.

Daren was a professional fireman. When he graduated with the rest of his training group of fifteen men, they agreed to celebrate by going sky-diving, and bought tickets. But one by one, for one reason or another, the rest pulled out. After some training in proper landing techniques, Daren was the only one of that group who turned up at Wilton early one morning back in 1994 for the great adventure. It turned into a great disaster. His parachute became entangled in itself. For about 2000 feet he was in free-fall, thinking it was all happening much faster than he expected. Landing with a crunch, he somehow managed to roll on impact as he had been trained to do. Horrified spectators rushed up and found him still conscious beneath the crumpled canopy. Mercifully, ambulances were close by, and Daren soon found himself in Liverpool Hospital. He remembered being asked at some stage whether he'd mind being airlifted by helicopter to the Prince Henry Hospital – "OK, so long as it does not crash!" he said – he'd had his crash for the day!

His spine was fractured and both long bones of his right leg were broken. But due to the spinal cord damage, there was no feeling in either leg. He appeared at that stage to be paraplegic. Daren was in hospital in plaster and traction for six months while the long bones of his right leg were healing. The bones of his left leg were not injured but the muscles did not work initially because of the fracture to his spine.

While the right leg was in traction, casts or splints to position the broken bones for healing, his left leg was just lying on the bed, as it seemed to require no special care. For many weeks he could not move it himself, but had to rely on the nurses. His left ankle stiffened in a bent position.

Over time and with physiotherapy some of the nerves and muscles recovered. Eventually there was enough function in both legs to enable him to learn to walk again, though he still had no feeling below the knees. He developed this characteristic 'rolling' gait. The right leg, originally so badly broken, was basically straight and functioning reasonably well. However, the left leg, which had become twisted at the ankle, was causing problems. Because he could walk only on the outside edge of the foot, and had no pain to warn him of trouble, this foot became damaged, ulcerated and infected.

Despite his injuries Daren had been able eventually to return to work with the Fire Brigade, on restricted duties. Over the next five years he saw a succession of doctors who tried many different treatments to heal the ulcer, but nothing worked – or not for long anyway. He'd had surgery, skin grafts, bone scraping and massive doses of antibiotics but the ulcer stubbornly persisted. Just before he came to me, a podiatrist had sent him to a vascular surgeon – doctor number 48, literally! – who had said that amputation was now the only option.

At that verdict, tough guy Daren told me he wept; he asked, "Isn't there anyone else I can see?"

"Well," the podiatrist said, "you could try the Fracture Clinic and ask for Dr Warren." So here he was.

I examined the foot and looked at his X-rays. I said, "Well, I am pretty sure that we can help you; but it is going to take a long time – at least a year of treatment. We'll need your complete co-operation." I explained that I had treated many patients with similar problems and that we were usually able to obtain healing of the ulcer. In addition, we should be able to teach him how to care for the foot and so avoid suffering a recurrence.

For Daren, it meant hope at last. Anything was better than losing his foot or part of his leg, or living with a permanently infected wound on his foot. I liked his determined, definite response. "OK," he said, "let's get on with it!"

And that we did, and I will return to his story in due course.

Daren is one of many grateful Australian patients saved from amputation because a certain English medical missionary, Dr Paul Brand, working in India in the 1950s with leprosy patients, used his common sense and realised that ulcers **will** heal if rested and protected. He was my chief surgical mentor – and a spiritual mentor too – a great man who died in 2004. The routine use of plaster casts to help heal ulcers has saved the feet of thousands, if not tens of thousands, of feet around the world.

Most Australians I have been able to help are relatively privileged patients, who, despite their misfortunes, could take the initiative to help themselves. On the other hand I have spent much of my life working, as Paul Brand did, with leprosy sufferers in the Third World. It was through helping them that I have learned the most. I thank God for the privilege of being able for over forty years to work as a medical missionary, a surgeon and physician. My work has mainly been in Asian countries, in Africa and the Middle East, but also in developed Western countries, including my own Australia – more countries than I care to count. It has been wonderful to be a part of a team bringing healing and the restoration of dignity, faith and hope to people who were often the most wretched and despised of all in their communities.

In 1959 I started work in Hong Kong with The Leprosy Mission, and now in retirement, I remain gratefully in association with that mission. By applying Paul Brand's principles and developing them further, I have been able to treat thousands of people with nerve damage and lack of pain perception from many different causes besides leprosy.

But how did I come to be doing this type of work? That requires telling the story of my crowded and complex life. I am now 77, and trying – not very successfully – to slow down and retire properly! In some ways I'd rather not do so completely, as each day brings new surprises and challenges.

It's a long story – I will start at the beginning.

2

Beginnings

My earliest recollections are of living in Cullenswood, near St Marys on the east coast of Tasmania, in an old rambling house – the Rectory. It was separated by an open field from the beautiful little stone church, originally built as a landowner's private chapel.

My grandfather, William Robert de Mey Warren had migrated from Devon, England in about 1880. He married Selina Jane Horrell in April 1884, and they had three children. The eldest, my father, Hubert Ernest de Mey Warren, known as Bert, was born in 1885 and educated in Melbourne. The family went to All Saints' Church of England, St Kilda, where he was a choir boy. From an early age he was fascinated by machinery and had a natural mechanical aptitude. It is said that he and a friend built and rode the first two motor cycles in Melbourne. He was apprenticed to a firm of marine engineers and later travelled overseas to work; on returning from a trip, he was invited to hear the evangelist George Grubb. That changed his whole outlook on life, as he became a committed Christian, with the motto *Jesus First.*

He became interested in mission work when a neighbour, Rex Joynt, went to the Roper River Mission Station in North Australia in 1908. Father entered Moore Theological College, Sydney, and was ordained in 1911 as a priest of the Church of England (now the Anglican Church of Australia). He was accepted by the Church Missionary Society (CMS) to serve among Aboriginal people in the Northern Territory at the incredibly isolated Roper River Mission on the Gulf of Carpentaria. He arrived there in June 1913 and that October, aged 28, became the superintendent, working with his friend Rex Joynt.

In 1915 the CMS decided that they required a boat for the work in the Gulf – so Bert Warren travelled south and bought an 18 foot craft and an engine to be installed later. Now his training as a marine engineer made sense – God knew what was needed. As skipper of the *Evangel* and later the *Holly* he voyaged some 10,000 nautical miles, including trips across the Gulf of Carpentaria taking stores from Thursday Island to the mission station at Roper River.

He had met my mother in Sydney at St Clement's, Marrickville, during his theological training. She was Ellie May Potter, a Sunday School teacher and trained school teacher. Both my parents were good with their hands – a hobby of hers was wood-carving – I guess that is where I get that gift. They married in 1914, and went together to North Australia to work among the aboriginal people for the best part of twenty years.

My father led hazardous pioneering expeditions to Groote Eylandt in the Gulf. He named its central peak Mount Ellie after my mother. In July 1916 at the Roper River Mission, their first child was born. Also called Hubert, he was always known as Bill – and was the first white child born in Arnhem Land. They returned to Melbourne in 1919 for the birth of their second child, Josephine. My mother and the children then returned to Roper River by sea, while Father and a friend undertook the 3000 mile (4,800 km) trip by car from Melbourne to North Australia via Queensland. This was the first time it had been attempted – an astonishing journey through a trackless wilderness. Even today it would be daunting. In the Gulf country a hidden tree trunk ripped out the sump of the car. Father made another from a kerosene tin and completed the journey. The aborigines called this car "little fella buggy run along quickfella no horse"! Father, who was very tall – about 193 cm (6 ft 4 ins) – they named "long fella cobberlili". Cobberlili was their name for a type of lizard.

In April 1920 tragedy struck. An epidemic hit the settlement – possibly the post-World War I influenza that killed so many. The sister I never knew, Josie, died aged thirteen months and an aboriginal child also died the next day. Bill, aged four, also became desperately ill. The whole station, black and white, met to pray for healing. Bill began to recover quickly and my parents were spared that double sorrow. But little Josie's death bonded them in a fellowship of suffering with their aboriginal friends, and this made a clear difference to their Christian ministry.

My parents did much to improve the lot of indigenous people in their areas and set up a home for the mixed blood children, the so-called "stolen generation". In that area at least, most of the children were unwanted in the aboriginal camps where their mothers lived and could not live with their fathers, mostly stockmen on the cattle stations. Instead of being neglected and rejected, these children were able to get loving care, schooling, health care and training for some sort of trade or service in the future.

My sister Helen was born in NSW in 1923, and my second brother David was born on Groote Eylandt in 1925 – again, the first white child born there. The children came south on slow voyages for schooling. Finally I arrived in 1929, born in Sydney, and I too was taken north to Roper River.

My father resigned from CMS in 1932 and took up the parish at Cullenswood. So we were together in Tasmania, the first time that our family had really lived together for any length of time.

It would be hard to find a greater climatic contrast. Tasmania was really cold at times. I remember Helen and David coming back from the fields one morning, carrying a great sheet of ice found down in the swamp. During the first "summer" that we were there, Mother asked one of the locals, "When does summer come?" "Well, it came on a Tuesday last year!" That was about it! But we were prepared for that. We had great open log fires and cooked on an open wood-range in the kitchen, and our lives centred on these places of warmth.

In 1933 my father was called back north for a very difficult assignment – to mediate in a dangerous dispute with aborigines at Caledon Bay, who had massacred five Japanese fishermen. Without allowing for possible provocation, a punitive expedition had been planned. But CMS proposed a Peace Expedition: a team of experienced missionaries with knowledge of the language and culture, to go unarmed to seek the facts and, if necessary, have the culprits brought to justice. The team my father Bert Warren led in 1933-34 seemed wonderfully successful in finding the truth. This whole incident made him quite famous. He then returned to his family in sleepy little Cullenswood. But later, to his distress, the Government broke its promises to the missionaries and to the aborigines who had surrendered to the white man's law.

We were a happy family. I cannot remember much of my father, except for some amusing incidents like the time he clapped his old hat on an echidna who had waddled into view during a family photography session. As rector of a parish, he was involved in his church work, and Mother assisted him ably. My elder brother Bill lived in Launceston where he was apprenticed – yes, you guessed it – as an engineer.

When my father was in northern Australia, the Bishop of Carpentaria broke a wheel of his car while visiting the mission. Darwin was hundreds of miles away over rough roads. Father, inventive as always, went off into the bush, came back with a suitable log of wood and *carved* a wheel that could be fitted onto the axle. Problem solved, the bishop drove back to Darwin. I was told that the bishop used that wooden wheel for quite a long time – said it was as good as a proper one!

I've inherited that gift of improvisation. I thoroughly enjoy "making do" and adapting and improvising things – something I thank God for. I gave myself great pleasure when I was growing up because I could make my clothes. Mother had taught me to sew at a very early age. In the war years when clothes were rationed I remodelled items from a late aunt's "glory box" to make clothes for myself.

In mid-1934, my father accepted a move to a suburb in Sydney. Mother was to take the children by sea with all the household goods, while Father would fly from Launceston to Melbourne on business, before travelling to Sydney. Father boarded the plane *Miss Hobart*, while we caught the steamer in Hobart for the trip to Sydney.

I can remember sitting on a staircase on the steamer. It was fun to be a five year old on a boat! My sister and I shared bunks in a cabin with my mother. Unlike my sister, I was not seasick, so I used to run around and pass things to her through the little portholes that opened from her bunk to the stairs leading up to the next deck. It became a great game.

I do not remember our arrival in Sydney. Nor do I remember that as the ship berthed, my Uncle Fred, Mother's brother, met us with the news that my father had been lost in the first Australian civil aviation disaster. The plane *Miss Hobart,* with its pilot and ten passengers, had gone down in Bass Strait and the wreckage was never found.

Several uncles, my mother's brothers, were to play an important part in helping us to settle as a family in Sydney. In November 1935, we moved into the house at Chatswood, where I still live. It was bought for us by the CMS, after an Australia-wide appeal, as a memorial to our father. It was indeed God's gift to us at that time. Without it, our family could have been destitute.

We soon became involved in the life of the local church, St Paul's Church of England, Chatswood – to which I still belong! – the youth fellowships, clubs and the Sunday School. Church became a very important part of our lives. CMS also had young people's groups which I joined. Mother often spoke at CMS meetings about the aboriginal work in which she and my father had been involved.

When old enough we three younger children became weekly

boarders, David at Trinity Grammar and the girls at St Catherine's School for Clergy Daughters at Waverley. This gave us a good mix – the discipline of a boarding school during the week, and family and church life and more freedom during the weekends. Our family life, so disrupted in the earlier years, was now much more stable, despite my father's death.

After she left school Helen studied botany and horticulture. From her I learnt a lot, and acquired my love of growing things – something that was useful when I worked in Asia. She also taught me how to embroider. I have fond memories of Mother, Helen and me sitting around the dining room table listening to the war news on the radio, embroidering things for her glory box. Helen did beautiful embroidery and insisted that when I embroidered, the back had to look as neat as the front. She little knew that she was training a surgeon to do nice neat work and tiny stitches, enabling me to reconstruct hands and faces.

The uncles were regular visitors as they came to 'fill in' for our father, taking us out for drives and bush walks. Big brother Bill, so much older, also took on the role of man about the house.

In my early teens I came to realise that just being brought up in a Christian family and going to church does not make someone a Christian. I determined that I was going to find out what God wanted me to do and to follow his leading. I started attending Crusaders – the Crusader Union youth organisation. Crusaders taught me that faith and trust in Jesus are of first importance and that I could never earn salvation by being "good". My outlook became different from that of most of the other girls at my school – despite its "clergy daughters" tag – as few had any real interest in following Christ.

I did make one very good friend – Kathleen Collett, who came to St Catherine's in fourth year high school. She was a boarder whose family lived on a property at Wee Waa in the far north-west of NSW.

I spent one school holiday there, and had a great time. I learned to ride a horse, and even had my first "surgery" lesson when I helped Mr Collett slaughter and cut up a lamb for meat.

Helen was clever and won many prizes, but I just managed to keep in the middle of the class. I still have a report from my senior years at St Cath's, stating that my writing and spelling were so bad that I would never pass the Leaving Certificate – but God obviously had other ideas! I certainly did not collect prizes, and never really made much effort to get to the top. That did not interest me. I preferred to play the piano and sing and sew and swim and do a little sport and gardening. I liked to play roles in plays and pageants and usually was in reading and voice production competitions. I well remember the King's Quotation as one of the pieces we had to recite in a competition in the war years:

And I said to the man who stood at the gate of the year:
'Give me a light that I may tread safely into the unknown.'
And he replied:
'Go out into the darkness and put your hand into the Hand of God.
That shall be to you better than light and safer than a known way.'

So I went forth, and finding the Hand of God, trod gladly into the night.
And He led me towards the hills and the breaking of day in the lone East.
From *God Knows* in *The Gate of the Year* by M. Louise Haskins

Eventually I had to determine what I was going to do when I left school. By this time, I knew that God wanted me to serve as a missionary, but in what profession? It was really a matter of talking to God and asking him to guide me. Whatever it was that I ended up doing, I prayed it would be the thing for which he had prepared and equipped me.

I did fail in my first attempt at the Leaving Certificate from St

Catherine's. For a second attempt, I went to Hornsby Girls' High School. That was very good for me because I met a very different group of girls, with a different outlook. Thanks to the coaching of my schoolmaster Uncle Fred, I improved enough in mathematics to scrape through the Leaving Certificate. I say "scrape through" because that was just what I did – I had just enough points for University entrance.

3

University and Beyond

My brother David and I both needed, and obtained, Commonwealth Scholarships to go to the University of Sydney. By the time I got there he had his first science degree, and was teaching at Geelong Grammar. He returned to Sydney University to lecture in chemistry when I was in my second year of Medicine. David gained his Ph.D. and eventually went on to win fame for the invention of the "Black Box" flight recorder.

Unlike David, I was not a good student – I'd never have got into Medicine these days – and at university I continued my undistinguished career. In the early years I had to sit for several "posts" – supplementary exams. Then I failed, and had to repeat the whole of third year. But the rest of the MB BS course caused me no real problems. I was into the practicalities, examining people and assessing their situation. I was able to use the practical streak I was born with, and work out the diagnosis by logic.

Leisure time during the university years was filled with the activities of the Evangelical Union (E.U.). I had many friends who were keen Christians and we attended Bible studies and meetings together. I also got a reputation for being able to cook for house parties, conferences, camps and beach missions. The latter were aimed at teaching Christian principles and bible stories to children and anyone who would come and listen. It was at a Childrens Special Service Mission (CSSM) Beach Mission that I first learnt to use a pressure cooker and sent a jet of stew onto the roof of the tent! Those were good days with wholesome fun and a lot of teasing amongst the members of the team.

The standard joke of the time was that CSSM meant 'Come single, soon married' – and I saw that happen many times, but never got caught myself. It was not that I did not have suitable friends – I have always been blessed with friends of both sexes with whom I could share my faith, my hopes, my work and my troubles. It was activities like these that helped me to learn to adapt what I had to meet any given situation. I learnt that if God asks me to do something, he has already provided what I need to complete the task – what I need materially, in strength or ability. Without knowing the eventual outcome I have learnt to trust him – and the results have been amazing.

People have questioned why I have never got married. "We live today, we dream tomorrow, but we only understand looking back." I certainly could never have undertaken the itinerant teaching program which God had in mind for me if I had had a husband and family. But in their place he has given me a world-wide family – young and old, of all nationalities and interests, people who are grateful that God had brought me to them to improve their quality of life. They have enriched my life, and here in Australia many of them welcome me as family whenever I come their way. I am forever grateful to God for this.

My other special interest was in music and singing. I played the piano and pipe organ for meetings and services if needed. I joined the church choir and the EU Choir and often went with groups to take evening services. Some of us used to sing hymns in a big hospital in Sydney on Sunday evenings and then go on to an open air service. I was told my voice could be heard over the traffic and several floors up even without a microphone. I am not sure if this was a compliment or a complaint!

During term I grabbed any experience available – one never knew what might be useful later. How else would I have known how to pack an autoclave?

It was sometime in the early 1950s that I attended an evening drawing room meeting run by the Christian Medical Fellowship.

It was advertised as a very special meeting. The guest speaker was Dr Paul Brand, from the UK but then working in India. He had us all mesmerised. He was talking about a new variety of surgery – new to us anyway. I thought he said that he moved muscles from one side of the arm to the other side to provide a function that the patient had lost. It took me a little time to realise that he did not move the muscle bulk but just transferred the tendon so that the muscle was given a new job but its nerve supply was not affected, so it would still continue to function. I thought little about it for the next few years, but this was to become a major part of the work God had for me to do.

In my early university years my married sister Helen was affected by a brain tumour and it was necessary for Mother to live with her in Victoria. Since Kathleen Collett's family now needed accommodation in Sydney, they moved into our house. Kathleen was doing nursing training at the War Memorial Hospital at Waverley. She completed three certificates and then went on to study at Bible college, as she too was challenged to move towards missionary work.

I sat my final examinations in 1953, graduating in January 1954. That year I was appointed a junior resident medical officer at the St George District Hospital. I got plenty of good experience in giving anaesthetics and in surgery and greatly enjoyed that side of my training. More recently there have been many more restrictions on what a junior resident can do, so the present trainees do not get nearly as much opportunity as we did in these specialities.

I needed to find a position for 1955 and applied for a surgical traineeship at several hospitals. I was notified that I was accepted to work in the Queen Victoria Hospital in Melbourne, and was thrilled as this was one of the few hospitals that had women surgeons permanently on staff. But they did not give me the job I applied for. On arrival there I found I had a routine obstetrics position. It was hard to accept that I was not going to do surgery. I did not know how valuable that obstetric experience was going to be in many situations in Asia. In those earlier days I really would have been happy to give up the obstetrics if I had not accepted that it must be God's plan for me.

In 1956, I became one of four registrars at Geelong District Hospital. One of my fellow registrars, Dr Ian Lyall, was also gaining experience for missionary work and we often worked together. At Geelong I gained an amazing amount of surgical, anaesthetic, and general medical experience. I learnt to lecture and to teach, especially the nurses. In January 1957 I was invited to stay and work in Geelong as a partner in one of the surgical practices. But I felt that this was not the life for me and so moved on.

My question then was: where next? Did I require further study or surgical experience, or was overseas missionary service the next step? It was clear that I was unlikely to obtain a true surgical training position, but I had shown that I could do many things if given a good written description of the procedure.

I decided on some language training and joined a Summer Institute of Linguistics (SIL) training course at Belgrave Heights, in the mountains east of Melbourne. Though it was fascinating, I soon learnt that I was not destined to be a linguist. I have no 'ear' for the fine differences in the way sounds are pronounced, words are said and tones produced. What I learnt still proved useful, but instead of completing the course, in March I began the post-graduate diploma course in Tropical Medicine and Hygiene held every year at Sydney University.

There were only about sixteen of us in that course, which dealt with most aspects of tropical medicine and associated subjects – safe housing, insect-proofing, the elimination of mosquitoes, provision of water supplies, food requirements – all necessary knowledge for those wishing to work in tropical countries. The course included statistics and we calculated our life expectancies. I in my twenties, was the youngest in that group of students, and female, so I was the only one thought likely to live to the year 2000! Well, I have done that!

But tragically one of the students, Norman Powys, a CMS missionary from Tanganyika, East Africa, married with three children, had a heart attack during the course and died the same day, aged only 38. The very moving funeral service in St Andrew's Cathedral was attended by all the teaching staff from the course. Some of the lecturers were very interesting and friendly people who would help me solve problems in later years.

The Christian Medical Fellowship to which I belonged had been investigating opportunities for an exchange medical program with Indonesia. Indonesian government medical officers would come here for training and experience, and in return Australians would gain experience working in Indonesia. This was a chance to use our medical skills in a third world situation, so some of us discussed the matter with an Indonesian attaché and lodged application forms. That was in 1957, and, to date, I have not received a reply! It was just part of our efforts to find the best way to use our ability and training in helping others and serving Christ. I was not surprised when another opening did come in an unexpected way.

Around July 1957, I was asked one day if I had worked at the Queen Victoria Hospital in Melbourne.

"Oh, yes", I replied.

"Were you doing Obstetrics and Gynaecology there?"

"Yes!" I affirmed.

"Did you do the premature babies?" The conversation was becoming more focused.

"Oh, yes, I did the whole thing," I reported.

"What are you going to do when you have finished your Tropical Medicine?"

"Well, I really do not know – I am knocking at doors. I am waiting for God to give the next lead and show me where I should go. Basically," I said, "I will go anywhere he calls me".

"Well now," I was told, "there is a hospital in South Korea that does obstetrics – it is the only dedicated obstetrics and women's hospital in the Republic of South Korea. The Australian doctor who is there at present is due to come home on leave. Her *locum tenens* has been hospitalised and cannot take up the position. We are therefore urgently in need of someone who can do the basic surgery and midwifery necessary to run this hospital, to relieve Dr Helen Mackenzie while she comes home on furlough."

Well, we live a day at a time, but often only understand by looking back. Here obviously was a purpose for that job at the "Queen Vic" which I thought was a surgical training job, but which turned out to be just an ordinary 'obstetrics and gynaecology' post.

I did not have a good reason for saying "No", so my papers were submitted. I am told that I was the most rapidly processed person that the Australian Presbyterian Mission had ever accepted for overseas service! Understandable, when it was only for eighteen months relieving Dr Helen.

And so when I finished my exams, I was busy trying to organise everything to go overseas. I had to get a passport. I had to buy clothes for Korea's cold winter. In Korea, I would be able to use Dr Mackenzie's blankets, sheets etc., so I did not need to take all that with me. However, I needed to raise more funds for various expenses, and so I organised a couple of short medical locums.

Since 1954 I had been driving a little black Ford Prefect car. It did yeoman service at the linguistics school, where cars were a relative rarity and was often overloaded with fellow students. It went by the name of "Alexander". The name came from one of A. A. Milne's children's poems:

"I had a little beetle, Alexander was his name
I kept him in a matchbox and he answered just the same –
But Nanny let my beetle out and beetle ran away! "

Up to this stage he had run away twice – once was when we skidded on a wet hill while crossing a bridge, and I landed on the railway line beneath. I was able to drive on. On another occasion Alexander got caught in sand drifts and ended up on his side. A couple of nice men came to the rescue and put him back on his wheels. Little did I realise when and how Alexander would run away again!

A few weeks before I was due to leave I was returning from seeing a patient on a night call. Crossing an intersection, my car was hit by a drunken driver and thrown onto a telegraph pole. I received just a few minor bruises but missed a meeting I was aiming to attend. Alexander was a write-off – but because of my insurance policy, the car was worth more that way than if I had sold it! So that solved the problem of when and how to sell the car! It helped pay my expenses – I could not have organised it better if I had tried!

4

Post-war South Korea

At Sydney airport on the 14th October 1957 I met Sister Cath Mackenzie for the first time. We boarded the plane en route to Korea. The flight took us via Darwin and Manila where we changed planes and boarded an American airliner. This flew us to Okinawa and then to Tokyo, just on sunset, which gave me the most beautiful photo of Mt Fujiyama silhouetted against the sunset sky. There we were accommodated in a hotel at the airline's expense – a rare bonus for me! Next morning it was back to the airport to board the flight for Seoul, South Korea.

I was fascinated by the scene below as we came in to land at Seoul. It was autumn; there were red peppers drying on the roofs, the fields were golden with grain, and the pine trees made a beautiful contrast. It was a lovely land to fly over. We landed at Kimpo Airport where some American Presbyterian missionaries met us, and took us by jeep to the domestic terminal on the other side of town. I was told to make the most of that piece of road because it was the best motorway in Korea! There were certainly plenty of potholes as Korea's roads had been badly damaged during the recent war, and very little had been done to repair them.

At the domestic airport our luggage was loaded, and we clambered on board a DC3 for the hour's flight south to Pusan. No sooner had we boarded, stowed our baggage and fastened our seat-belts, when they announced that there was a typhoon coming up. The flight was cancelled, so we climbed out again. Fortunately our American friends were still at the airport, and they raced us back to the city, and instead of a flight, secured some tickets on the night train to Pusan.

These were sleeping carriages, with three tiers of bunks across the carriage. There was precious little head or leg room. As Koreans are relatively short, whereas I am 5 ft 8 ins (1.74 metres) and Cath Mackenzie was about the same height, neither of us could stretch out properly.

Quite a number of the staff from the hospital greeted us at the station at Pusanjin when we arrived. We were taken up the lower slopes of the mountain to the hospital which was situated in the Australian Presbyterian Mission compound.

The hospital was founded by Cath and her sister Dr Helen Mackenzie. Brought up in Korea where their parents Rev & Mrs James Noble Mackenzie were missionaries, they had returned to Australia in the 1930s, Helen to train as a doctor, Cath as a nurse. In 1940 they too had headed for Korea as missionaries, but the ship had to turn back, as trouble lay ahead. Cath and Helen were advised to return home. Korea, at that time ruled by Japan, was certainly off-limits for the duration of the war. Remarkably determined women, within a short time they were on their way to China instead. They flew in from Calcutta "over the hump" – the Himalayas – as the Japanese had occupied a large part of China. These intrepid women set up an obstetrics hospital in the mountains of south-western China. There they worked for a couple of years in what was originally an old temple. They laughed about the fact that they literally kept their gold, their only practical currency for supplies, "in the lap of the gods"! The "god" of the temple was curtained off from the rest of the floor space where the patients were housed.

By the time they left China, the Korean War was retreating up the peninsula. The Mackenzie sisters were among the first foreigners allowed to return to Korea in 1952. Initially, they set up their hospital in another disused temple on the lower slopes of the mountain behind the port of Pusan. The American Army was, of course, well established in South Korea after the Korean War. They were very helpful assisting in general projects and built a number of hospitals 'to order', including one for the Mackenzie sisters. So now they had a building in which to establish their women's hospital for obstetrics, gynaecology and paediatrics.

The area was still extremely crowded. Thousands of refugees from North Korea had come south and settled on the hills behind Pusan. They had built makeshift houses, swelling the town's population. Helen and Cath established the Il Sin Hospital (*Il Sin* means 'New Day') to meet the needs of these women. At that time Korean women usually gave birth on the floor at home. People slept on the floor, not on beds as we know them. If they were fortunate, they might be attended by a midwife. Otherwise, a relative took care of the delivery. Very rarely did they go to hospital, unless complications developed.

Here in these crowded conditions, it was hardly ideal to have a baby at home, but that was what continued to happen. However, once the hospital was open, a continuous stream of women came regularly to the ante-natal clinic to be checked while they were pregnant, and also for delivery. We did have a lot of complicated cases, patients who had travelled for many hours over rough roads in some sort of vehicle. Not only were we trying to deliver babies and save the lives of both mother and baby, but we were also trying to train the midwives. It was a busy hospital and there was plenty to do.

I arrived at the hospital on October 17th, 1957. There were several 'Welcomes' for me, but these were combined with 'Farewells' to Dr Helen, who was taking her holidays in Australia a few weeks later. The staff was mostly Korean and were really very capable. The senior Korean doctor, Dr Lee Hung-Chu, had asked for another foreigner to come and work with her while Dr Mackenzie was away. There are times when it is much better to be able to blame the foreigner if something has gone wrong or has not been done in the desired way – after all I did not understand Korean! I soon learnt to read it phonetically however, so I could read the names on the charts, etc. At least Korean is a relatively easy language to read and write.

Dr Lee was very good at diagnosis and surgery. Quite often I would give the anaesthetic or supervise one of the Korean doctors giving an anaesthetic, while Dr Lee did the surgery – a good reason for the experience I had gained in Melbourne in 1955-56. Dr Lee and I worked together; we alternated our nights on call and our weekends as well, though normally I would work Sunday mornings so that Dr Lee could attend the church just up the hill. I attended the service sometimes, and was reprimanded once because I put my money into the collection with only one hand! In Korea one always gives or receives anything with two hands. And one bows when greeting anyone. Just some of the traditions and customs one needs to learn for each different country.

There were all sorts on interesting breaks in our routine. In spring we enjoyed the masses of cherry blossom in the neighbouring park. During the eighteen months I was there, I was able to visit various other parts of Korea and attended the Christian Medical Fellowship conference in the autumn, meeting medical workers from many different countries.

The patients were very grateful for what we could do to help them. Many of the women were very young, with complications during pregnancy or childbirth. Without the hospital they would probably have died. Some had suffered past injuries ("fistulae") through obstructed labour and were leaking urine. It was a tremendous joy to them to realise that these awful injuries could be surgically repaired, enabling them to lead normal lives and to be accepted in their communities. I did some of these operations. It was this type of work which so endeared the Christian hospitals to the local people. Korea today has a high proportion of Christians and many can point back to contact with hospitals, schools or colleges as the factor in introducing them to Jesus.

Medicine as we practised it in Korea was a far cry from what I had been taught in Sydney, but I could not have asked for a better introduction to third world medicine, where we did not have all the laboratory facilities and senior consultants to assist. In Australia we were taught that when making a diagnosis, one needed to have one and only one, cause for all the patient's symptoms. A single diagnosis however often did not fit our Korean patients. Many of them would have several diseases at once. Typhoid was often with us, and tuberculosis was always with us. One very ill patient had toxaemia of pregnancy causing seizures, but also tuberculosis, meningitis and typhoid fever – all at the same time. She recovered! Often all that was needed was basic simple nursing care, and very few of the patients who came to us died. Most went home with healthy babies.

Many were anaemic but one learnt how to adapt one's treatments. Blood transfusions were expensive, unreliable and often did not really supply the correction of the anaemia that was desired.

For medication we had to import many drugs and it took 6-9 months for an order to return to us. So we bought what we could locally. In obstetrics one needs a lot of intravenous fluids and the only ones we could buy were badly contaminated. We managed to get a still from the American army to distil water, and I then taught the pharmacist to mix the medications and the maintenance man to sterilise the intravenous fluids.

Later in the year an Australian pharmacist visited and was very interested. "Oh", she said, "have you tested its sterility?" I looked at her, questioning. "Yes," she said, "you inject the fluid into the ears of white rabbits, and watch the reaction." Where did she think I would get white rabbits – out of a hat? "No, we haven't", I replied, "but we get far fewer reactions when we use this for the patients than with the fluid from the market!"

The hospital also provided care for women missionaries working in Korea. We became very friendly with some of them and visited their places of work. One of these was the new work of The Mission to Lepers that had recently been set up in Taegu. The English nurse on their staff, Miss Grace Bennett, became a very good friend, whom I saw and stayed with many times over the next forty years. On some of my visits to Taegu I went out with her to help in leprosy outpatient clinics. This was my first introduction to the care of leprosy patients.

One of the sad and difficult things about being a missionary far from home, especially in the 1950s and earlier, before flying became commonplace, was when a crisis struck at home. While I was in Korea my sister Helen, six years older than I, died. It was just not feasible for me to return home.

Towards the end of my stay there we entertained a visitor from the UK, the general secretary, Mr Miller, of the Mission to Lepers. He had come to film some of the leprosy work in Korea. There was a big "leper colony" near Pusan, founded many years before by Helen and Cath Mackenzie's father, and one day we took the English visitor and other staff members there. Before he left Mr Miller asked me if I could go and do a locum at the leprosy hospital in Hong Kong. As I had no definite plans and was waiting for God's direction, I agreed to go. I planned to leave Korea when Helen returned, take a month's holiday in Japan and then travel on to Hong Kong to arrive there in May 1959.

5

Hong Kong – First Impressions

I arrived in Hong Kong from Japan on Sunday morning, 4th May 1959, by sea. I remember being enthralled with the whole vast moving panorama of that beautiful harbour, bustling with boats. It is still much the same, though Hong Kong at that time was relatively undeveloped.

Our ship, the Kamboj, moored in the middle of the harbour between the island of Hong Kong and the Kowloon Peninsula. Victoria – the city on Hong Kong Island – was the administrative centre for the region, and there The Leprosy Mission International (TLM) (though in those days it was called The Mission to Lepers) had its office. Opposite, on the Kowloon peninsula waterfront, was the large Post Office with the YMCA close by. The Star Ferry linked Kowloon and Victoria.

The Reverend Jim Waddell, the administrator of TLM hospital, met me. He had brought a mission launch in to meet me and my trunk and we set off for the hospital on the island of Hay Ling Chau. When the weather was good, the boat trip was enjoyable. Over the next fifteen years however, I often felt decidedly seedy on that trip, and would do the trip horizontally. But on this first voyage, everything was interesting; the weather was nice and I did not feel squeamish at all.

Hay Ling Chau literally means 'The Island of the Happy Spirit', but we called it 'Island of Happy Healing'. 'Hay Ling' means happy spirit, and the Chinese word 'chau' refers to an island in the estuary of a river. It is situated seven miles by sea from Victoria.

The island, the Government Leprosy Institution, was leased to The Mission to Lepers. It was almost as an act of desperation that the

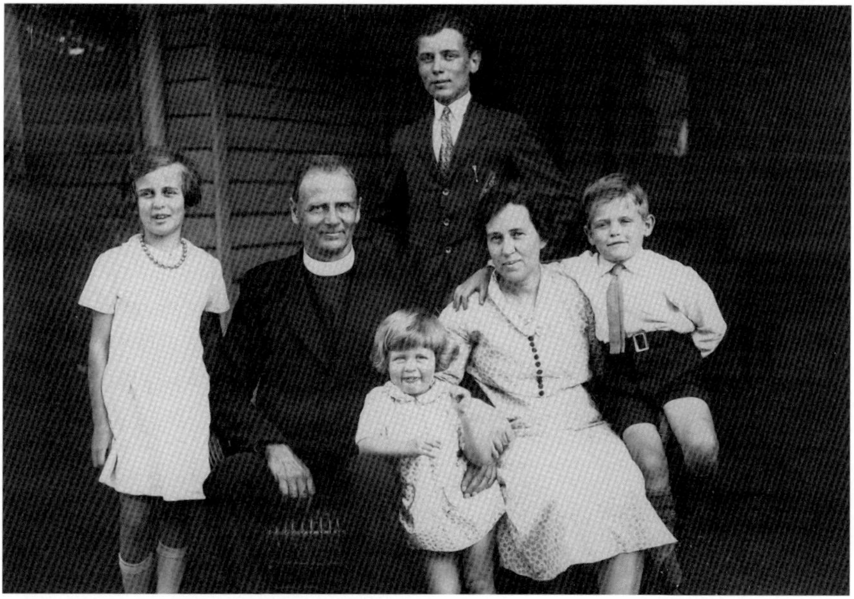

The Warren family - Cullenswood, Tasmania 1934
Helen, Father, Grace, Bill, Mother, David

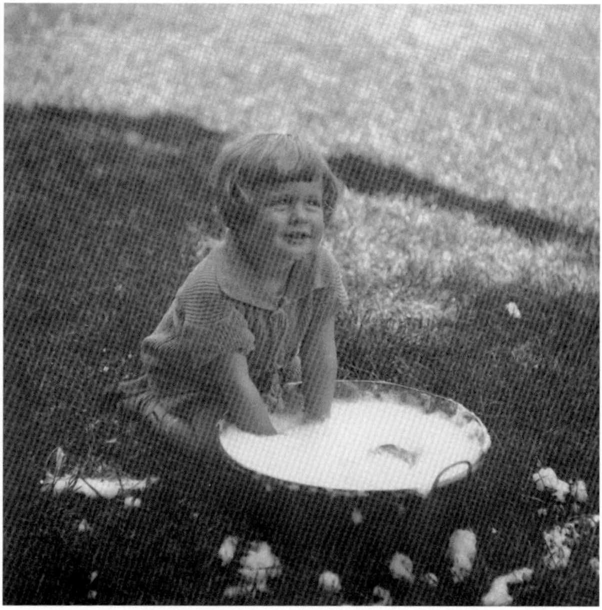

Young Grace scrubs up – aged 3

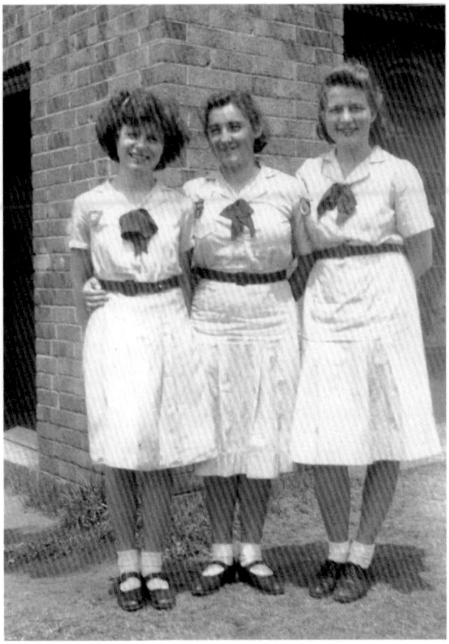

Grace (right) with Kathleen Collett (centre) and another school friend, 1944

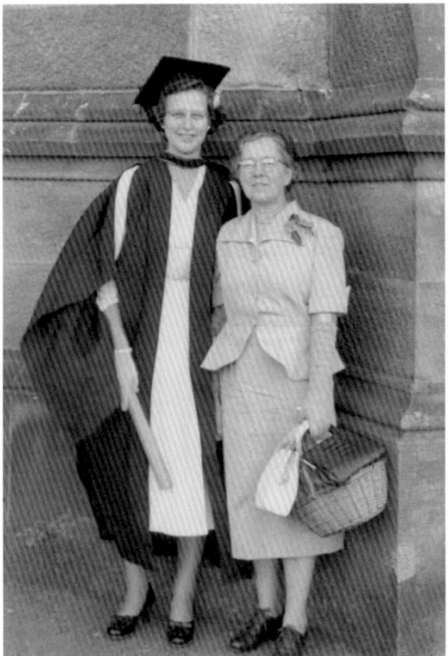

Graduation - Doctor Grace with mother (Ellie); Sydney University, 1954

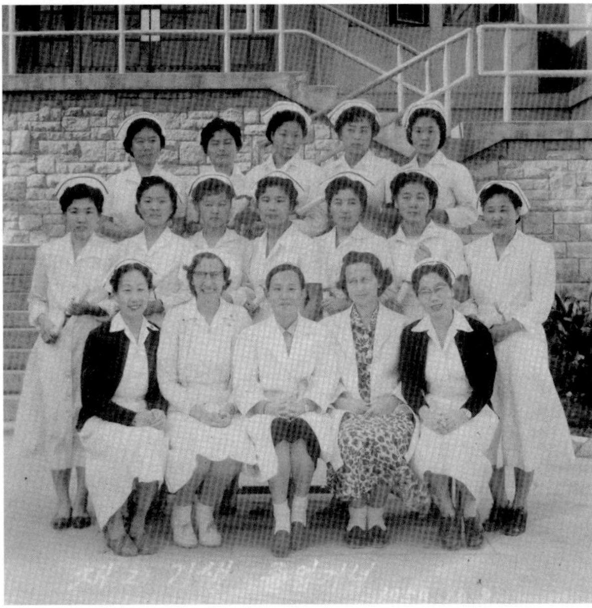

Sister Cath McKenzie, Dr Lee Hung-Chu (Centre front) and Dr Grace with graduating nurses at Il Sin Hospital - Pusan, Korea

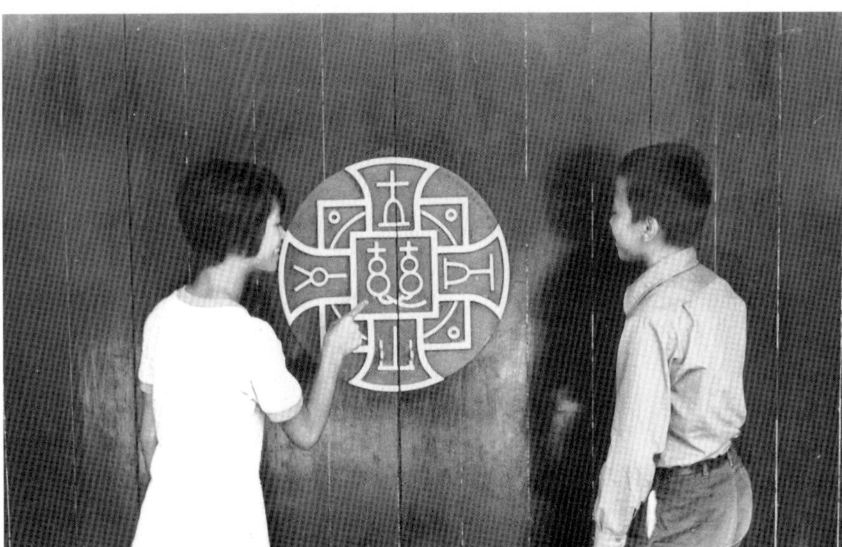

Brass symbol of Hong Kong TLM auxilliary

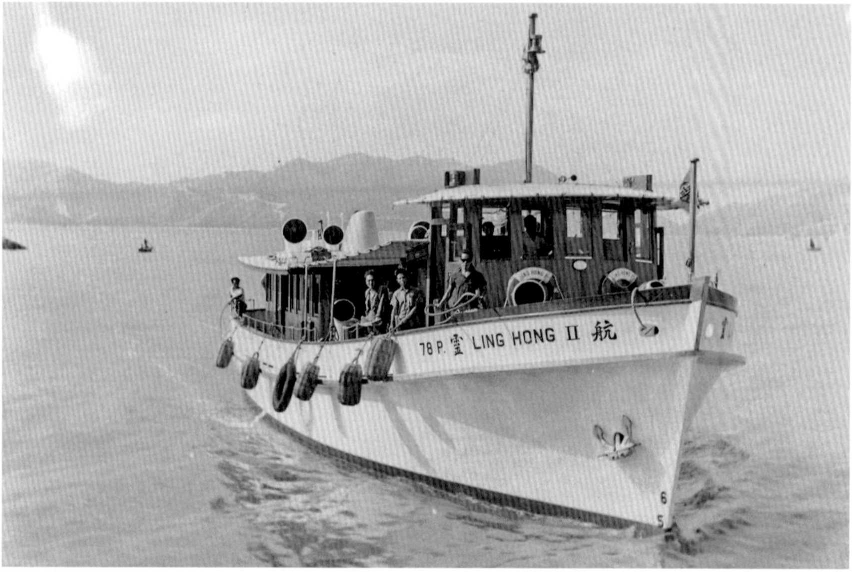

The 'Ling Hong' - The main launch for supply and transport - Hong Kong

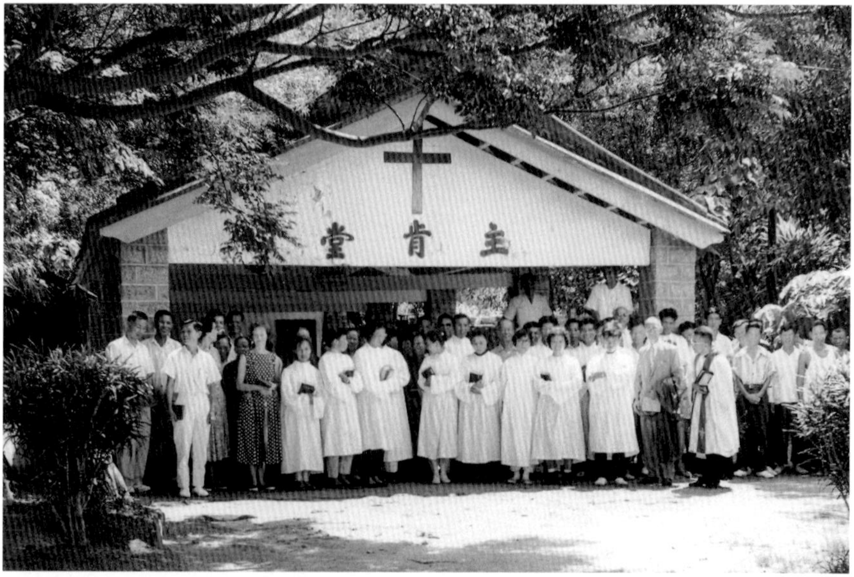

Choir and members of 'The Lord is Willing' Church Hay Ling Chau - 1964

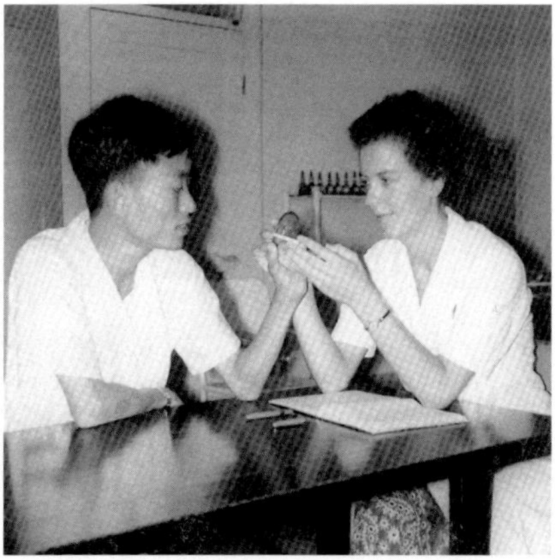

Jean Watson, physiotherapist - checking finger angles and function

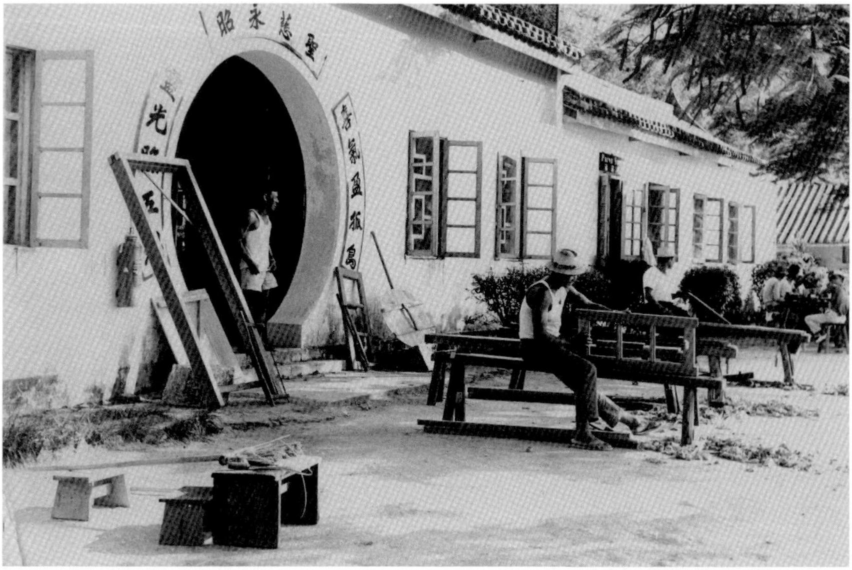

Inscribed Moon door feature of the beach front carpenter shop

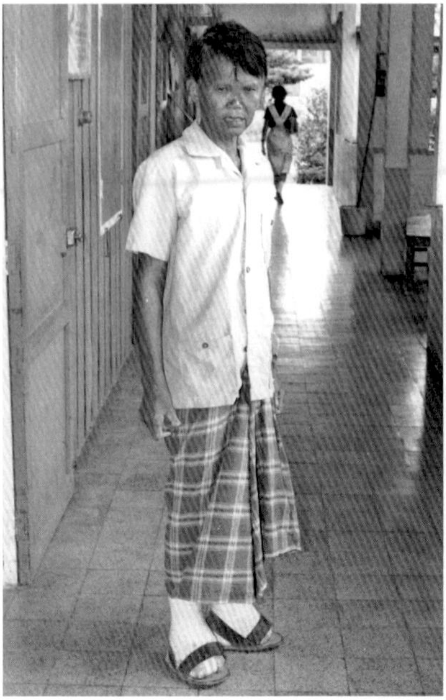

Despite ulcers, this patient can walk in two plasters: his ulcers will heal while in the casts

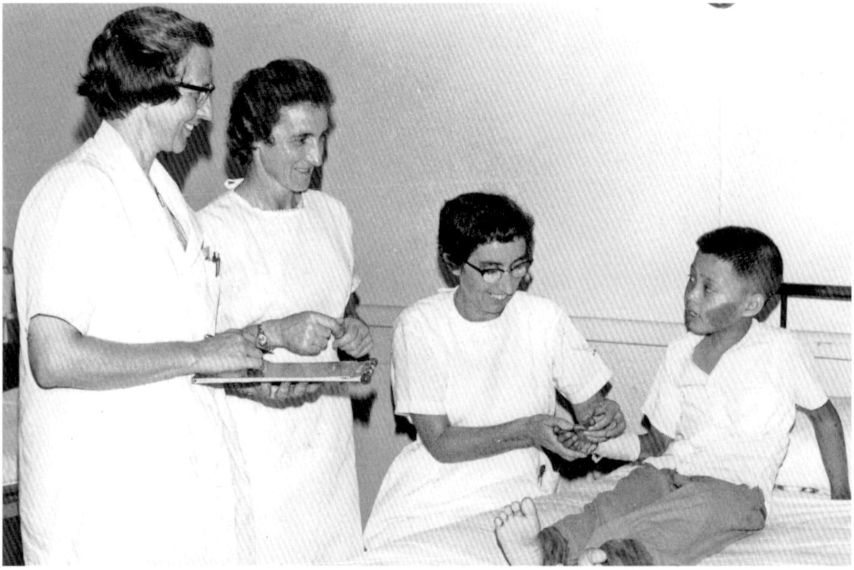

Small boy with a typical facial skin lesion, attended by Dr Grace, Sr Kath Collett, and Sr Joyce Ledger - Hay Ling Chau, Hong Kong

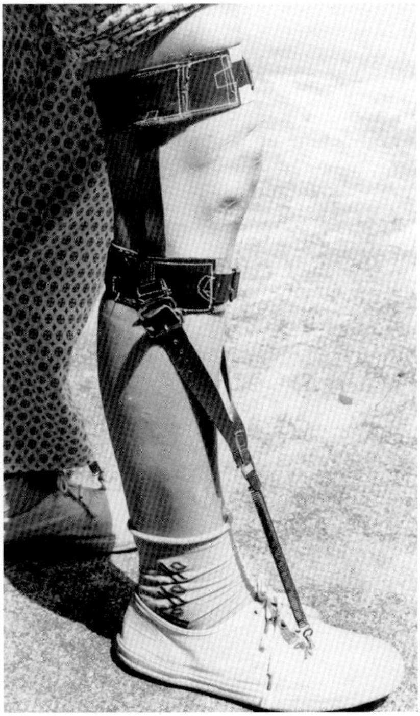

Foot drop spring, facilitates walking with paralysed foot, in early stages of treatment

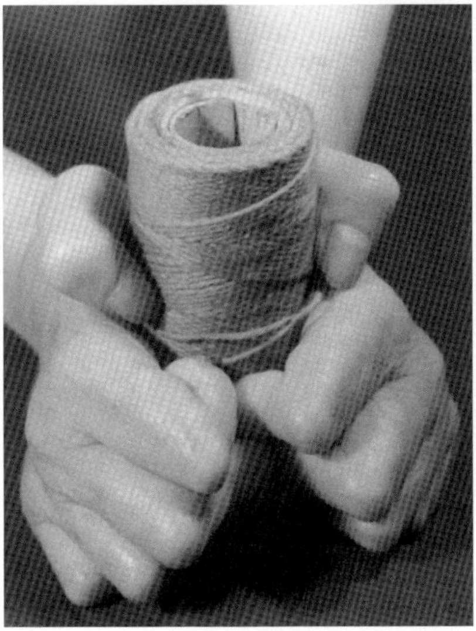

Typical 'clawed hand' deformity showing problems of grasp

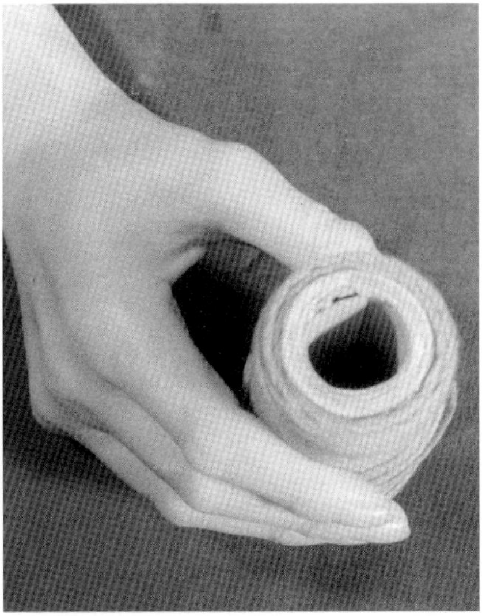

Ah Sum's clawed hand after reconstructive surgery

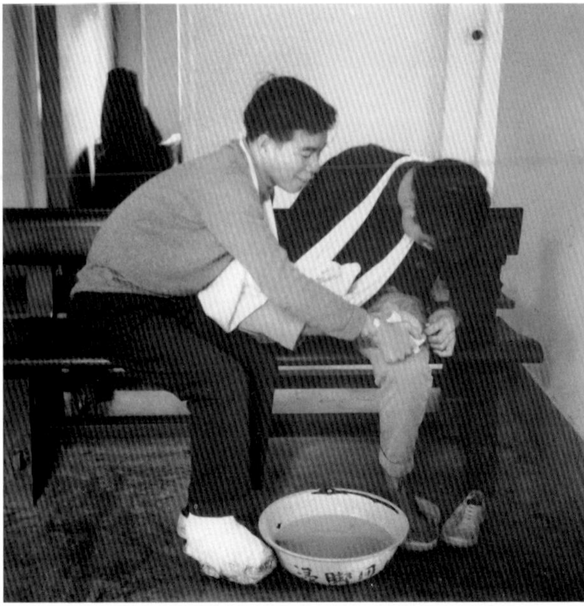

Two patients helping one another, doing self care - Hong Kong

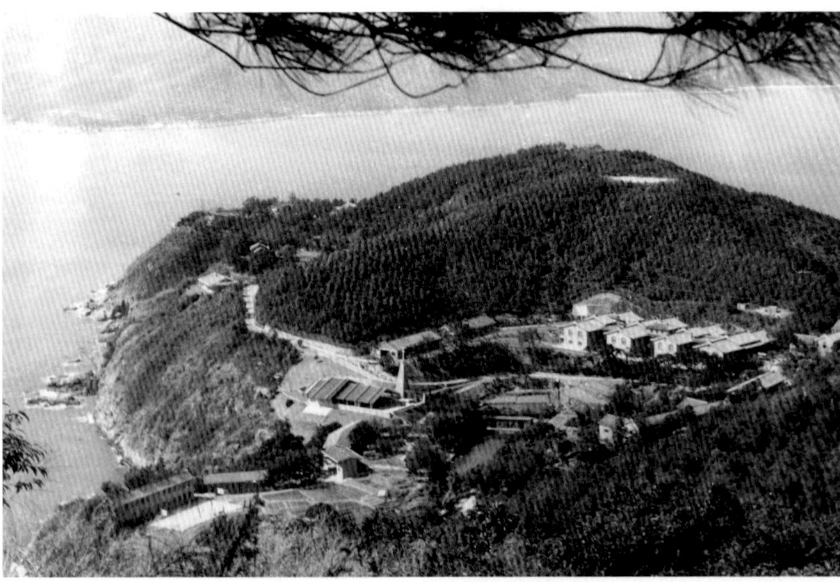

Hospital block, church (with spire), patient and staff cottages, helicopter pad, and reafforested hillsides in main valley at Hay Ling Chau

Government selected it for the development of a leprosy hospital in the early fifties. Large numbers of patients needing treatment were in temporary accommodation at Sandy Bay on the main Hong Kong Island. They got their medicines from government outpatient clinics, but many of them were homeless and needed all-round care.

Dr Neil Fraser, an Englishman who had worked in China with the Presbyterian Mission, had set out to try to find a place that was suitable for a leprosy hospital. He combed the hills, looking for somewhere with arable land and preferably its own water supply – a place where he could build a hospital with reasonable facilities for a largish number of patients to live long term. Local villagers fearful of leprosy opposed any suggested sites. So eventually this almost uninhabited island was designated. It was used occasionally by fishermen, but lacked a good water supply. In fact, Dr Fraser said, it had none of the facilities that he wanted for a leprosy hospital.

In 1952 it was still accepted that leprosy was a highly infectious disease and that segregation was essential, usually for life. However, by then the drug dapsone (DDS) was leading to some patients being discharged cured. And the work of missionary doctor Paul Brand in India to prevent deformity and to correct the disabilities was changing attitudes to leprosy. I had heard Paul speak when I was a medical student and later I would work with him. (See chapter 11.)

Some patients had been taken from Sandy Bay to the island in 1952, physically able men selected to help with the development of the island. There was a need to construct buildings and start the farm work. Twenty years later, some of those men said that they had literally destroyed their hands and feet in building Hay Ling Chau, quarrying the stones, building, mixing cement, laying stone and digging gardens. In the 1950s, the full impact of leprosy-related abnormalities of pain perception was not recognised. These men were damaging themselves while working and were doing little to treat the wounds or to prevent the trauma. People believed the wounds and sores were a part of leprosy. Today we know they are not and can be prevented by adequate care.

Dapsone had been introduced as an effective drug treatment in the late 1940s, but its effect was slow and it did not seem to help the dreaded deformities. It would be another twenty years before it was appreciated that dapsone made a person non-infectious but that the deformities had other causes. People needed to realise that the infection of leprosy was, in fact, not the major problem. The greatest problem was that, once this germ was established in the body, the patient's own immune system attacked the nerves and other tissues in an attempt to eliminate the infection. In so doing it destroyed some nerves and took away the ability to feel pain – to feel anything at all, in some cases.

Leprosy is often considered to be a skin disease. It is far more. It is really a systemic disease with skin manifestations. It can involve other systems. The effects on the nervous system are the most serious. Motor nerve damage is the most obvious, when muscle weakness occurs and some muscles are paralysed, resulting in deformity and abnormality of function. Sensory nerve damage causes abnormalities of sensory perception. This may not sound serious but its results are the most far reaching, especially the loss of pain perception. Leprosy-affected hands and feet become very prone to injury. But patients commonly say, "It does not hurt – it does not matter!"

Eventually it became accepted that leprosy patients, even if uncomplaining, must not be expected to do heavy labouring work without adequate safeguards. By the time I got there, a team of non-leprosy labourers we called the 'healthy workmen' were carrying out any heavy or rough work needing to be done on the island. There was much else, however, that patients could do.

Hay Ling Chau was in the forefront of the trend towards modern leprosy treatment centres. Dr Fraser intended to make it a model for future work and planned that the patients who came would all be trained to do something. If they already had a skill such as cooking, gardening, building or tailoring, then they could probably continue in that capacity. But if they had no skill, they would be able to learn one. The occupation of each patient was actually part of the treatment. In many places the attitude was: "Oh, we are poor unlucky lepers – now you have to take care of us." Dr Fraser's approach was: "You *can* work!" "Where there is a will there is a way!" And in most cases this was true. Hence, he was years ahead of his time and we sought to improve the ability of every patient to realise their potential.

That first day, Jim Waddell took me on foot for a tour of the island, three or four hills connected together. I saw the hospital, patients' cottages, the pine forest, the reservoir. And on top of the hill nearest to the hospital was a helicopter landing site from which we could evacuate emergency medical cases. That was where we held the Easter Dawn Service each year.

I remember tramping over the hills, exploring and finding lovely orchids. Jim Waddell was rather surprised to find that I knew something about water supplies, catchments and reticulation – from our Tropical Medicine course. I was always interested in the 'big picture'. We called lots of things GMT (Good Missionary Training)! I still teach students, "There is nothing you can learn that won't be useful for something other than the purpose for which it was originally intended."

The patients all lived in standardised accommodation – granite houses with simple bunks in small dormitories. Conditions, spartan for anyone used to middle class comfort, were well above the average standard in Hong Kong at that time. There were kerosene stoves for cooking. We had to teach patients how to cook safely – all part of the training for living with hands with abnormal pain perception. They had to learn to work and cook without injuring themselves, or, if they did get a cut or a burn, what to do about it.

I moved into one of the simple but rather attractive two bedroom stone cottages on the other side of the hill. To get to the Visitors' Centre from my new home, I would walk along a path which twisted and turned around the hill and through the pine plantation – a pleasant walk that took only a few minutes. At night one certainly needed a torch – it was not a smooth concrete path. Beryl Batstone, a nurse from UK, shared my house, perched on a cliff with lawn between our front veranda and banana palms and pawpaws on the cliff edge, which fell quite steeply to the sea. We could watch the fishing boats far below and hear drums being banged to frighten the fish into nets. A patient helped tend our garden. We grew fresh vegetables and I had an orchid plot and lots of flowers.

Further down the road from our place was the Marine Police Post – a government-occupied building on a point overlooking our jetty, a good vantage point for observing harbour activity. Silvermine Bay lay opposite, and Lantau, one of the larger islands. On its high hills were cottages where some Europeans spent their summer holidays to escape the heat at sea level.

In Hong Kong in summer, the 7 am news often told us the temperature was already 85/90 degrees F. (27/35 degrees C.) with 98% humidity. We would arrive at the hospital after our ten minute walk to get there, wringing wet with the exertion of walking in that heat and humidity.

In the evenings we were grateful for cool sea breezes. But the summer nights were long, hot and sticky. There were electric fans until 10 pm when the generators went off; then we'd try to sleep under our mosquito nets. One night I remember the amah, our house help, coming in calling my name anxiously. It was dark and I found a torch. She had got up to go to the bathroom with a small torch and had found a cobra there, coiled around the water pipe. With my larger torch I was able to lure it outside. A few blows from a big spade left it writhing on the concrete path.

If there was need at the hospital we could get the generators turned on, but normally we managed with kerosene lanterns. There was not really much on at night! Thank goodness – the days were long and busy enough.

All our supplies came from Hong Kong by boat. In many respects the island was an idyllic sort of place. But understandably many patients did not like being separated from their families. Others had long been separated anyway; they were in Hong Kong alone. They had managed to get out of China in the hope of finding treatment in Hong Kong, or sometimes had left China because life there had become too difficult. These patients had nowhere to go if they left us, and some had marked deformities and faced social ostracism. Hay Ling Chau was their only home and their refuge.

About 500 patients lived there in 1959; our maximum in the mid-1960s was 543. From the start, patients had been coming and going because, once we stated they were non-infectious the government allowed them to leave Hay Ling Chau. Originally, the government wanted everyone in Hong Kong with leprosy to be treated in our hospital. But with 4,000 to 5,000 patients on their books, that was impractical and most were non-infectious anyhow.

The island's boat, the *Ling Hong*, was normally moored at the end of the island's long jetty, with the smaller launch, the *Hay Ling*, tied up alongside. At weekends, early morning and evening, there was always a line of patients sitting on the wharf fishing.

The *Ling Hong* made the trip to Hong Kong most days of the week. On Saturday mornings, it would call into Victoria and pick up new patients at 8 am. The Government doctors did not just send them from the clinics – the patient had to agree to come; there was no compulsion. Nor was there any obligation to stay if they did not like the place or the treatment we offered. The Hong Kong Government paid the mission so much per patient. Other funds came from TLM supporters around the world.

New arrivals were allocated one of the cottages. After their medical conditions had been properly assessed every patient capable of working was allocated a job to do. Some would be admitted to Hay Ling Chau's lovely hospital, with about fifty beds.

Across the road from the hospital's main entrance was the workshop where patients did various handcrafts. One was embroidery. Those with bad feet could sit to work and, if necessary, could have their feet up. In Hong Kong, there was a tourist market for embroidered articles such as those made on the island and so embroidery could provide a future occupation.

One of my many jobs later was keeping an eye on what the patients were doing, not only at the craft workshop but all over the island. They needed work suited to their handicaps. Leprosy patients worked as ward aides, nurses, plumbers, cooks, cleaners, gardeners and in animal husbandry. Our electricity generators were manned by patients. We had gas stoves and kerosene refrigerators. It was a busy working community, mostly self-sufficient.

Near the hospital was the school. Some patients had been school teachers, others we co-opted into teaching. For my medical and surgical work too, everything was well established. The operating theatre even had an air-conditioner. Later on, a new physiotherapy room was built with space for all the needed equipment – pulleys, ropes and parallel bars for practising walking.

We were very much aware of the problems of drug addiction. We occasionally admitted drug addicts for withdrawal, on condition they requested it and signed a pledge not to take any more drugs – at least not while with us. More easily said than done, of course. Once, the new patients included Ah Yuen with tuberculosis and a history of drug addiction. When questioned, "Oh," he said "I have given it up." I warned him that we would not permit it. "Oh, no problem," he insisted, "I have given it up." So I warned the nurses to watch carefully, for we usually found telltale bits of the silver paper that came wrapped around the drug.

Ah Yuen had arrived on the Saturday morning. On the Monday at 8 am the nurse told me that they had found silver paper on Sunday. I said "OK – put him in a wheel chair and bring him across to the morning clinic." Monday's clinic was always busy. He arrived, I greeted him and he said he was OK – so I said I just needed to give him a little injection. I gave it to him in the arm in the sight of about 50 others waiting to be seen, while he sat there – all smiles to start with. However the injection is one that rapidly neutralises the opium. Within ten minutes he was rolling on the floor suffering the agonies of sudden withdrawal. Now everyone on the island knew I could tell if someone was on opium! That fixed Ah Yuen – we never had trouble from him again and for a long time the number of drug incidents amongst others dropped significantly!

Life on the island moved at a regular pace. During those early days I must confess I was not very enthralled with the job. Over 500 patients, all with chronic problems; and in those days we could not offer them a lot of optimism about their future. A doctor needs to feel that his or her work counts for something and is making a real difference in people's lives. Initially I was far from sure I was going to enjoy this job and find it worthwhile. I had only promised to serve for 18 months, so for that time at least I needed to stay and learn the ropes.

6

Learning the Ropes – Language and Leprosy

On arrival at Hay Ling Chau, I had a lot to learn. Leprosy was a totally new sphere of medicine for me, one in which we had received very inadequate training.

When I did my first clinic and met the patients I knew no Chinese, so my interpreters were patients who had learnt English on the island. I was working with Dr Douglas Harman, the English doctor who had been in charge since Neil Fraser returned to England. Doug taught me what he had learned, medically and surgically. He also used to lecture visiting medical students, a job which I inherited.

But that first day was a bit hairy! Without the patients interpreting I wouldn't have been any use at all. But I began to get a 'feel' for leprosy, for what the patients needed, and what could be done. On that first day, I think my basic vocabulary was the Chinese word *"ho"* which means 'good'. I soon learnt that *"Ho"* in Chinese also means Yes, and *ho ho* meant very good and *ho di* meant better! *'M Ho* means *NO!* with this vocabulary I was soon known as the "Ho Ho doctor"! If you say "*Ho 'm ho?*" it means "Are you good or not good?" In the morning, you say "*Nay ho mah*" which means, "Are you well? Are you good?" So with one basic word, at least I could be polite. But I soon learnt a few more words like 'pain' and 'every day' and words for what the patients needed to do and so gradually I gained a little of the essential vocabulary.

However it was a slow process and I have never become fluent in any of the Asian languages that I work in. This has its advantages. When I go into a hospital to teach and I cannot speak the local language, I have to be provided with an interpreter, who is often the doctor. I cannot do the clinic alone. Hence he watches me at work and I can easily judge by the translations he gives if he really understands the question and its reply! Very useful.

The basic language in Hong Kong is Cantonese, named after the city of Canton (Guangzhou) some 70 kilometres inland. It had developed as their trade language. Many of the Hong Kong people could also speak Swatow or Chujow. Today most of the young people who come from China to Australia have done their schooling in Mandarin, and those from Hong Kong and the south also speak Cantonese. I had some lessons in Cantonese but I did not do very well. The fascinating discovery I soon made was that, no matter which dialect is used, all Chinese people can read and write the same characters because the characters represent ideas, not actual spoken words or sounds.

In the first few weeks I learnt a few phrases that we needed for everyday work. There were lots of words similar in sound but of very different meaning. After a while, somebody pointed out that I had better be a bit more careful in using the correct tone. This really became obvious later in Thailand when I was informed that I kept asking patients if they had been in the priesthood instead of "Do you have pain?" – rather odd when I asked the women that question as well as the men!

In the mornings, Dr Harman took the more complicated medical clinic and I had the "ulcer clinic" to which a less complicated group of patients came. But they still needed their basic leprosy medication. Initially this was dapsone and was given twice weekly. However, even in 1959 there were patients who did not do well on that basic dose, so we were trying other medications as well in combination with the dapsone. We kept excellent records so it was relatively easy to check the progress and the effectiveness of the drugs.

Most of the patients who came to us in the active stage of the disease had leprosy bacilli that could be found in their skin, and our laboratory technician Mr Yip, a former patient, was an expert finding them and keeping me notified of progress. He could tell if the numbers of the bacilli were decreasing or if there were signs of drug resistance. If the patient was not definitely progressing towards healing we could introduce some other medication. We also had to examine them on admission to see if there were other diseases that needed to be treated, because otherwise the leprosy was not likely to respond to treatment.

For most patients the progress to healing was slow and steady. The more severely affected patients stayed five years or more, the milder cases for shorter periods. A few only stayed a few months, especially those who just came for rehabilitation surgery. After leaving us they continued to get medication as outpatients in Hong Kong and to take their dapsone at home. They needed to be followed up for years. Later I had to re-admit some patients who had tried to stop treatment too soon and had relapsed. Or perhaps the bacilli had become resistant to the dapsone and so they needed other drugs. This contrasted sharply with the previous leprosy routines that involved admission for life.

I did not need to do all the dressings myself for those attending my clinic. Patient medical orderlies, or dressers as we called them, did that. I did have to look at the wounds and check their progress, and keep records. Initially, many of the patients were walking around on ulcers which were dressed regularly in the clinic. If the ulcers were really bad, the patient was admitted to hospital for complete bed rest. There we had little "trolley seats", four wheeled stools on which the patient could sit, resting one foot on a bar and using the other foot to propel it around. Using the trolley seat the patient was able to go to the bathroom and out onto the lawn and across to physiotherapy without walking on the affected foot.

But in the early days we were not nearly strict enough about insisting that wounded feet were really rested and protected. In leprosy centres it was generally accepted that ulcers were all part of leprosy. They might be operated on, with even part of the foot being removed. But a few articles were beginning to appear in the literature as to how to save these feet and prevent amputation. To begin with I just accepted what was being done at Hay Ling Chau, and slowly changed my methods as I observed results.

I soon learnt that these ulcers would heal with certain types of dressing and management, and that other things were a complete waste of time and money. With staff we discussed how to get wounds healed in the quickest possible time. I soon learnt a major lesson, that it is not so much the dressing that is placed on the broken tissue (i.e. on the ulcer) that heals the wound, but the way the wound is protected from further trauma. A patient with poor perception of pain on developing a blister on a foot will happily keep walking, whereas a person with good sensation would limp or remove the shoe to prevent friction. These ulcers needed to be rested and protected to enable the tissues to heal. This discovery was to play a very important part in my work in the future. It was reinforced by Dr Paul Brand's work, and I soon discovered the advantages of using the plaster casts that he had introduced into leprosy care as an effective means of healing ulcers.

I also realised how much footwear affects the incidence of ulceration and its healing. At that time, Japanese thongs (with a strap between the two biggest toes and no heel strap) were very popular, especially in third world countries. But they were the wrong sort of footwear for patients with neuropathic (nerve-damaged) feet. There was no means of keeping them on the foot. On many occasions I saw a patient walk down a path and leave the thong behind without realising it. Not good for an anaesthetic foot that needed protection! So relatively soon we started insisting that patients must not wear the thong type of footwear at all. They must have a shoe that protected the foot and would not fall off easily.

There were plenty of inexpensive canvas shoes on the market. With laces done up properly they did not fall off, as long as the heel was well into the shoe.

We had our own shoe maker who would custom-make shoes to suit problem feet. We recommended gym boots (lacing above the ankle) for some, or canvas shoes with special resilient insoles that we provided. With proper care there was less chance of their destroying their hands and feet. Having them work while with us helped them to see what they could do without putting their limbs at risk. Unfortunately "good" leather shoes were often too hard in the soles, and also the leather uppers rubbed and could cause local pressure and ulcers on the top (dorsum) of the foot, especially the toes. A good thing about the canvas tennis shoes was that the patients could keep them on when they went fishing or collecting shell fish. Rock or coral cuts on anaesthetic feet could be a menace.

In those days I had a remarkably good memory for any rules I had made. Woe betide the patient who deliberately did something against my orders! One warm summer's day I was lecturing the medical students in the small tutorial room off the laboratory. The window opened onto the main road where patients were walking up and down on their daily routines. I was facing the window and the students faced me. They were startled by my sudden yell, "Ah Song, where are your shoes?" I had seen a patient whom I had specifically ordered to wear proper shoes, walking up the road in thongs. He heard me through the open window and was highly embarrassed. He knew I would be with the students and had not expected me to detect his "crime"! I am afraid I took a delight in catching the patients out doing things they were told not to do. One of the patients' names for me was "the Old Dragon"! (I was in my early thirties.) The reason I needed to be such a dragon was that these things were so important if they were ever to get better – and stay better.

Once a week we used to show a film out on the lawn at the back of the hospital, and all the patients, including those in hospital, could go. On occasion I took the opportunity to sneak round in the dark and check on the patients. Who was wearing the wrong shoes? Who was not wearing the sling I had ordered to protect an arm that needed rest? Who was walking without crutches when they were told to use them? Who was out and about when they had been told to stay in bed? When I caught them, it was very good for their discipline, to help teach patients they must learn to care for themselves.

Even in Dr Harman's mainly medical clinic we insisted that feet be checked, as many patients could not feel if they had damaged their feet. One Monday the children were all up for their weekly dapsone dosage. The boys had had a lovely time at Scout camp. As each child came through I insisted, "Shoes and socks off!" I looked at Young Ma's foot and there was a red patch on the ball of one foot. It felt a little hot, and swollen. I asked, "What have you been doing?" "Oh, nothing special." He'd been racing round the camp all weekend. "Oh no, I did not go without shoes." But maybe they had not been properly laced up and had been slipping, for he had a real friction burn on his foot. This spelt danger. If he was allowed to continue to walk on that foot he would have an ulcer by the weekend. So for him it was "Into bed in hospital!" No walking, full bed rest, not even allowed to go to the toilet as that would mean putting weight on the foot. We put a splint on the foot to protect it from bumping and friction. By the weekend it had completely healed – no redness, no swelling and no discomfort. So he was allowed back to school on the Monday. I do not remember any more trouble with his feet.

Many patients were sent to me because of non-healing foot ulcers. One such patient – Ah Yung – was about 25 years old on admission. He had cut his heel on a piece of coral years before. The ulcers persisted and the infection had destroyed part of the heel bone. On admission he still had a gaping hole on the sole of his foot and yet he arrived happily walking on it. No pain! Well, that was the last time he walked on it for many months. We put him into a special plaster cast to give the tissues a chance to heal. The ulcer did heal over and the bone infection cleared, but the shape of the foot had altered so much that more ulcers would develop as soon as he walked on it. We operated and reconstructed the foot and then put him into a plaster cast for nine months. At the end of that time he had a foot that was reasonably normal in shape and on which he could wear a normal shoe.

One of the patients who came regularly to my clinic was one of our school teachers, Miss Chu, who had been a teacher before she developed obvious signs of leprosy. When I met her she was probably in her early forties with very badly deformed hands. She certainly was no longer infectious but needed our help for her foot and hand problems. She had already lost half of each foot and she had chronic infections and ulcers as well. We operated on both her hands and her feet over the years and we managed to improve her function and keep her feet free of ulcers, though she always had to wear special shoes to protect and preserve what was left of them. As she was quite plump, there was quite a lot of strain on her feet. But once we developed our improved foot care program she really learnt to look after herself and had minimal problems in later years. She stayed with us for years, teaching the children in the school and playing an important part in Bible teaching. Eventually she married one of the ex-patient staff.

7

Life on Hay Ling Chau

Good staff are vital to the smooth running of any institution. On Hay Ling Chau we had some excellent people such as the matron, Mrs Lee, a qualified nurse and midwife who trained in China in a mission hospital before escaping to Hong Kong. She usefully spoke several dialects, and besides being Head of Nursing she also acted as the pharmacist, making up and dispensing the medicines to the patients.

Mr Ho was the Chinese administrator, also a pleasant and capable fellow. He had been a pilot in the Chinese air force and was so trusted that he had flown one of the last planes out of China before the Japanese took over, taking valuable documents into Hong Kong. He was an excellent organiser who could see what needed to be done, and could see through the patients' tricks and wiles that we had to contend with at times.

On Mr Ho's office walls were boards, one for each of the cottages where the patients lived around the island. Each board had photos of the patients living in that cottage and there were several boards for those in the hospital. Every patient on admission had an identity photo taken and was allocated a number. This was so convenient if you were looking for a patient and did not know the name or admission number, as you could look around and find the photo. So many of the names were similar that I could not keep track of them, and I knew many of them by their numbers. That's not un-Chinese, as people are often called "Brother Number 3" and so on! The photographs served another good purpose. If I did facial plastic surgery, we had the record of what he or she had looked like beforehand.

A few patients were chronically dissatisfied – patients who felt that they shouldn't have to work. They expected to be looked after. This is where Mr Ho was excellent. He would explain to them, yes, they were in hospital, but since they were not actually sick they could do something useful; there is nothing more boring than just sitting around doing nothing. Not many refused to cooperate, but we were fortunate in that there was no compulsion to come to us for their treatment. This meant that we could insist on some work for the institution. If the patients were not prepared to work at all, we could just say "Goodbye"! That usually settled it. They'd stay, thank you! Life was much easier on Hay Ling Chau than in Hong Kong – especially if they showed some obvious stigma of leprosy.

There were three or four Chinese nurses. As well as Cantonese, each spoke a Chinese dialect, Swatow, and they had all come out from China. Some of them had husbands and children in Hong Kong, so they lived with us during their working week and travelled backwards and forwards on the *Ling Hong*. From time to time Chinese doctors also worked on the island. Many of these doctors stayed for years and proved very useful. Dr Zia had been an army doctor in his younger days and was very good, and Dr Lam, who was a keenly committed Christian, stayed with us for many years.

We taught the nurses, and the patients whom we called 'dressers', who had been trained in simple first aid and nursing, to sterilise the equipment they used as required. Throughout the hospital we sterilised all that was needed for the dressing round every day.

Staff included Dr Doug Harman and his wife Gladys. That first year, Gladys did a lot of work, sorting gifts of clothes and medical supplies as well as looking after their three children. When Doug and Gladys returned to the UK we welcomed Dr Stuart Goodwin, a younger man who came for one tour of service and then left us to go into pathology. Having trained at Karigiri in India before reaching Hong Kong, he brought with him some new ideas and techniques which he passed on to me.

I have already talked about working with Jim Waddell who was Administrator when I arrived. Later Alan Waudby with his wife Rena, a qualified doctor, and their three children came to replace Jim. They had worked in West Africa. They moved into the Harmans' house, although Rena later stayed in Hong Kong with the children for their schooling. Occasionally she was able to help us medically.

One of the jobs that the staff had to share was showing visitors around the island. It was frequently the expatriate staff who did this, unless the group was Chinese-speaking.

I inherited from Dr Harman the responsibility of teaching leprosy to the medical students from the Hong Kong University. The only medical school in Hong Kong at that time was at the University of Hong Kong. A group of about five or six medical students at a time would come over and live in one of the stone houses that we kept especially for them.

From Monday morning til they left on the Friday midday boat we had a steady stream of lectures and demonstrations for them. One could give them a good grounding and experience so that they would really know something about leprosy. We would get them to examine patients, write up their studies and do all the usual things. In Hong Kong, in 1959, there was still a great fear about leprosy, especially amongst the Chinese. Tradition has it that most students wore only old clothes while with us and dropped them off the back of the boat on the way back into town, not wanting to take the infection home!

Because of this excessive fear, I felt that this experience with leprosy was a very important part of their training. When they first came to us, they would say frankly: "No, I've never seen a leprosy patient. Oh, no, I've never touched one!" So I had to be very firm with them while teaching, calling them up one at a time, and making them do a full examination, so that they actually touched the patients – but not before I had explained that these patients were on effective treatment and therefore not infectious at all.

The students were thus introduced to leprosy, and many realised that they had probably seen and dealt with leprosy patients before without realising it. I often say that one usually only finds what one looks for. As they had not been taught about leprosy, they were unlikely to look for it. There were some duplicated notes on leprosy given out, but they did not cover all the problems that we were dealing with. So over the next few years, I rewrote them and made them into a respectable volume dealing with leprosy – its appearance, classification, treatment and the management of complications. Every medical student that came got this reference handout. They knew that there was often a question on leprosy in their final examinations.

A few years later, the University of Hong Kong decided to follow the lead of medical schools in the more developed countries: students would not need a whole week of leprosy instruction. Leprosy was dying out and other diseases needed more time, while psychiatry and mental illness needed more emphasis. They planned to eliminate completely the students' visits to Hay Ling Chau, but I wangled a compromise whereby I would go into Hong Kong at the beginning of their clinical year and give them two hours of basic theory in their morning lectures. They would then spend one day on the island and would be able to see the clinical patients and what we were doing for them. I called a roll on that day, and, unless a student got ticked as attending, he or she would not be allowed to sit for exams! It continued that way for all the years I was in Hong Kong until Hay Ling Chau closed.

My early experience in Geelong had prepared me for teaching these trainee doctors. In my travels I have met some of them, now working in other centres. A common statement would be: "Oh yes,

I know you, Dr Warren – you taught us leprosy at Hay Ling Chau!" But I am afraid they did not catch the 'bug' to specialise in leprosy, because we never got anyone from Hong Kong who wanted to come and work at the leprosy hospital. The doctors sent to work with us were ones who had trained in China and who were granted only a provisional medical registration.

At the weekends I stayed home on the island. Somebody had to be available and on call as we always had some sick patients. Usually on a Saturday afternoon we would have visitors to tour the island. Tourists, church workers, medical people and others who wanted to see the place. Whatever their reason for coming, most were amazed at the extent of the work and how much we were doing to transform hopeless lives and to make them useful and productive. By using basically simple procedures, carefully carried out, we could completely change the outlook for the patients. These methods were affordable anywhere in the world where leprosy was a problem.

One day Beryl Batstone was in the background of a group that was being shown around by one of the staff, and noticed that instead of listening, a visitor was sticky-beaking to see what was behind screens in the wards. "What's behind that screen?" he inquired.

"Oh," she said, "That is the man Dr Warren did a full face lift on yesterday."

"Face lift!" said the man with astonishment. (In the 1960s face lifts were highly specialised and rarely done.) In no time he was back with a group to hear all about it. Granted, I had not done the type of face lift he might have been thinking of, but nevertheless we had greatly improved the appearance of this patient's face.

And so day by day I continued my routine work. Life was very full but very orderly.

On Sunday mornings we had a service in the little church. It had no walls – just a roof resting on brick pillars. The Chinese characters on the front translated as '*The Lord is Willing*' *Church*. The name comes from the Bible story of the healing of the leper who came to Jesus and said, "If you will, you can make me clean." And Jesus said, "I will; be clean." The name was a reminder to patients that Jesus would help them too, if they asked him.

Many patients came to that church. In latter years, the Chinese pastor was Mr Leung Sing Sang, but there were others before him. I used to check on anyone that was sick in the hospital and then go down to the church. There was an old pedal organ and a patients' choir to lead the singing. My place was on the organ seat. Here again was a use for skills picked up earlier. As a teenager, I had learned to play our church's pipe organ and played sometimes for Sunday School. But here there was a pedal harmonium organ, so I enjoyed myself pedalling away while I played and sang! That was another part of the whole ministry. At that time there was no one else on the island able to play.

Later, a lovely new church was built with proper walls and glass windows looking out over the mountains and the sea. There was an electronic organ then, which was very nice to play; I continued to be the organist.

A number of patients were baptised. When asked why they wanted to become Christians, many of them said things like, "Well you are the people who have come to look after us. Our religion does not really have any respect the way you do for people who have leprosy. They treat us as outcasts. But you have come from overseas, you care for us, you give us medical treatment. In what you are doing we can see that God cares for us." And so for reasons like these they wanted to be baptised; they too wanted to be Christians. Some of the pastors and helpers were extremely committed to looking after the patients and helping them to cope with the problems of their lives. They helped them learn to trust and follow Jesus, so that they could serve him and show his love in their own communities when they went back to them.

To quote Stanley Browne's book, which in many ways sets out the principles of the mission, "Although The Leprosy Mission is avowedly Christian, and evangelistic, yet its policy allows for no discrimination against patients on any grounds whatever – of creed, race or colour. No pressure is exerted on patients to listen to the Christian message, but the Mission insists that, in its own institutions the Christian Gospel should be preached and exemplified for all to hear." [*Leprosy – New Hope and Continuing Challenge*, 1966]

Quite often, patients became staff members. Mr Yip, an excellent worker, was the laboratory technician. He was in his twenties when he came to us for treatment, was reasonably well educated and spoke English. He had a usable claw hand, which had been operated on before I arrived. He could not feel heat or pain, but was able to do his work, though part of it entailed using a bunsen burner. He learnt how to look after his hands – and not to hold hot test tubes in his fingers! He was always ready to show off to visitors the increased function that the surgery had given him.

Mr Yip was able to do the pathology tests for leprosy and became a real expert. Many a time in other Asian countries, I have wished that I had him working with me. One of the problems of leprosy is to know exactly how severe the infection is. A reliable laboratory technician can estimate of the number of bacteria in a skin smear, giving a much better picture than clinical examination alone. One can then assess how much treatment is going to be needed and how long it should continue.

By contrast, one of the other ex-patient staff members was forever having problems with his hands and his feet, which also lacked pain sensitivity. But unlike, Mr Yip, he did not care for himself. I constantly had to chase him up to check on his feet to see if he had ulcers and if he was doing his exercises. When we did operate on his hands, he was not prepared to exercise, to try to maximise the function and to keep them mobile and useful. This was such a pity because these Hong Kong patients, even as early as 1959, had advantages that many of the other leprosy patients of the world had yet to receive – rehabilitation surgery plus physiotherapy, that could remove the stigma of the disease and give them hands, feet and faces that were functional and socially acceptable.

Initially, physiotherapy was done in the outpatients' waiting hall, by a therapist who came over a couple of mornings a week. I had to learn a lot of it myself, especially for those who had had surgery. When the casts came off I had to teach the patients what I wanted them to do. Later on the women's support group of the Hong Kong Leprosy Mission raised the funds to provide an excellent physiotherapy building.

In late 1960 Jean Watson, a physiotherapist trained in UK, joined us. She had spent time in India en route learning the special techniques. She was expert at the exercises which were needed for both pre- and post-operative leprosy patients. It was marvellous having Jean in charge of the physiotherapy. She trained some patients as her assistants. Mr Leung Kwai Fong was highly skilled and motivated and spoke good English. He would find patients who needed treatment and get them started. He and others could do most of the work even when Jean was away. This was important later, because once I took up visiting Malaya (later Malaysia) on a regular basis and Jean followed me to do the physiotherapy, the men at Hay Ling Chau ran the physiotherapy department.

With our Malaya and Singapore trips Jean started her own travelling ministry that would eventually have a much wider influence than mine. She taught the physiotherapy of leprosy in Australia and Africa as well as Asia, and, as I write, she is still in Asia running prevention of deformity programs. She was awarded the OBE (in UK) for her many years of service to leprosy sufferers.

8

Hay Ling Chau Patients: Hope and Despair

Leprosy is not an inherited disease. Nor is it caught from a mother who is having adequate treatment. In Hong Kong in the 1950s research showed that children born to families in which one or both parents had leprosy did not develop the disease if the parents were on regular treatment. Eventually this fact became well accepted. But a small baby would be very vulnerable if breast fed by an untreated mother. Live leprosy germs are secreted in the breast milk, and the mother can be coughing and sneezing leprosy bacilli over the baby's face. If a mother or other carer is receiving adequate treatment however the germs are killed rapidly and the child will not catch it from them.

It has been internationally confirmed that it is rare for a husband to catch leprosy from an infected wife or vice versa. Usually both partners would not have it unless they had met and married as patients. That was of course quite a common occurrence because of the stigma of leprosy. In many countries, leprosy patients were not allowed to marry people without leprosy. In an early stage, when the disease was hidden, a marriage might take place, but once the spouse found out, that was quite often the end of the marriage. At Hay Ling Chau we did not have any married couples both with leprosy, so one parent generally stayed in Hong Kong with any healthy children.

Three children from one family were with us at one stage, each with leprosy: a girl aged nine, a boy aged six and a girl aged four. The father did not have leprosy, but we discovered that the mother had died when the baby was small, with an unknown skin condition, so we assumed that she had had leprosy and passed it on.

All children on the island went to school up to the age of sixteen. A trade apprenticeship could follow, or other work that had a future in it. So they could reach a reasonable educational standard, whereas they might have missed out altogether if they had remained at home. Patients who had formerly been school teachers were in their element and we made good use of them.

One patient, Ah Sum, was admitted with very deformed hands. In his late twenties, he had been a professional hand-knitter. When he came to us, his hands were a mess and he could no longer manage his needles. I could not see much future in his knitting, so we started him off on another handcraft. We taught him to embroider table cloths and towels using a large frame. Then, even with his bad hands, he was capable of pulling the needle up and down through the material to make patterns, flowers and other designs. So during the day, he worked in the embroidery shop. This embroidery, when complete, was washed and ironed by the 'healthy' laundry staff (not by patients) and would then sold in the craft shop.

Meanwhile, Ah Sum was taught how to care for his hands with physiotherapy, exercising them every day till he was surprised at how much mobility returned to them. Then came the big day for the first surgery. We operated on the fingers of one hand first, and then, a couple of months later, the other hand. Then we corrected the first thumb, to give him a proper pinch and grip, followed by the second thumb, so that eventually both his hands were functional.

Ah Sum still managed to do his embroidery. Even though his hands were in plaster after surgery, the thumb and the fingers would not be immobilised at the same time.

He stayed with us for a couple of years and was very grateful, because eventually he had hands which looked like hands. His fingers were no longer stiff and bent and knobbly and were usable. Above all, he could knit with them once again. He could be seen working in the embroidery shop all day. Later, if one wandered around in the twilight of a summer's evening, he could be found rapidly clicking his knitting needles as he worked on into the night. He usually knitted on a big circular needle so that, if he was knitting a sweater, it had no seams at all and was knitted beautifully. I had no idea how fast he could knit until one day Mr Ho, the administrator, said that Ah Sum had asked if he could please knit something for me. After discussion I purchased enough thick teal-coloured five-ply wool to make into a cardigan for my elder brother. I conveyed the details via an interpreter – my Cantonese was never good enough for that sort of thing.

On a Monday morning I gave Mr Ho the wool and some buttons for Ah Sum. On the Friday afternoon there was the cardigan finished and waiting for me on my desk – beautifully knitted without a seam in sight! Ah Sum had been working in our embroidery shop every day, and yet had found the time to produce a man's cardigan in less than five days of his spare time. After that he decided the time had come for him to leave us and return to Hong Kong to resume his knitting as a business, supporting himself and his family.

There are many others about whom we could tell stories. One day in the mid 1960s a remarkable man, Mr Lum, hobbled off the launch. All his possessions were in a rucksack on his back: this was the only way he could carry them, since he had mere stumps for hands, with neither fingers nor thumbs. An old hat jammed on his head partially hid his face. He preferred people not to notice that he had no eyebrows and had burnt his nose. Yet he was irrepressible, constantly joking with fellow passengers and, was obviously already on good terms with the other new arrivals.

He had been living alone in a shack in someone's back yard, supporting himself by gardening and doing odd jobs but injuring himself frequently in the process. The owner's wife had objected to the smell from the open wounds and ulcers on his hands. In order not to be driven away from the shack, his only home, he had chopped off the offending fingers with an axe. Horrifying as this seems, leprosy's nerve-deadening effects meant he did not find it painful. His hands, feet and face were all affected. By the time he arrived at Hay Ling Chau his hands had virtually healed and certainly did not smell; but how does one cope without fingers!

Mr Lum had learned to cope in unique ways. He could strike a match by holding it between his teeth and the matchbox between his two hand stumps. But a match had flared up and burnt the tip off his nose. Hence the hat he wore to shade his face and hide the burns. He was also trying to hide the loss of his eyebrows, a stigma which immediately suggested leprosy in its most severe form. In addition he had multiple ulcers on his feet and had destroyed most of his toes. That was why he walked with such an unusual gait. So for ulcer care, I ordered that he be put straight into a hospital bed.

Yet we knew that as far as his leprosy was concerned he was now a burnt-out case. Despite his appalling disabilities and somewhat repellent appearance, he would not give the disease to anybody else. People naturally shunned him however because of his deformities. Mr Lum, we learned, had only been living in Hong Kong for a few years. He had left his village in China because the local inhabitants, for fear of his leprosy, had threatened his wife and children. He was not allowed to use the village well and the family too was likely to be banned from using it. Eventually, for their sake, he had decided to leave home for good and fled to Hong Kong. After some months there he had got a friend to write and tell the family that he was dead. But here he was with us, alive and remarkably cheerful in the face of his sad history and multiple disabilities.

We set to work to clean up the foot ulcers. We taught him self-care to help prevent new ulcers and provided suitable shoes to protect his feet from further injury. When the infection had been controlled, I operated on his hands. Without fingers or thumbs, all he had left were the long bones in the hands – what we call the metacarpals, five of them on each hand. I removed the second one in such a way that he could use the first, the one that originally belonged to the thumb, to pinch against the third, the long finger one. We called them lobster hands – not a pretty sight, but functional – and that is what this man needed.

After surgery he was able to hold objects such as a spoon with one hand to feed himself. He also learnt how to weave and make table mats and do various other types of handcrafts. Mr Lum regained a degree of independence and self respect. He could now do something useful and was no longer completely dependent on others. For a number of years he lived with us on the island, and, like many others, became an occupational therapy aide, teaching others how to make the most of their disabled hands and to do handcrafts. Few can better teach, train and encourage others than one who shares their disabilities or even has far worse ones. In time, by means of grafting, we also gave him a new pair of eyebrows. The fact that he had a scarred nose did not worry him as, unlike the missing eyebrows, that was not a known stigma of leprosy. With eyebrows he would find more ready acceptance when he eventually returned to Hong Kong.

There was also Mr Wong, again with multiple leprosy problems. He had very bad hands and was completely paralysed in both feet below the knees. When he walked, you could hear him 'plop, plop, plop', as one foot after the other slapped down because he had no muscle to control them. We corrected the foot-drop on both feet and then worked on his hands. One hand was easy – a routine fingers and thumbs job. But the other hand required inventive surgery because there was only one working muscle. We managed to transfer tendons so he ended up with a hand which still looked like a hand and with which he had some grip. And somehow he managed to work with skill and competence as a weaver.

He too had no family that we knew of in Hong Kong, but he was always ready to help anybody else with a deformity or a disability. For a number of years, Mr Wong walked in the Fifteen Kilometre Walk to raise funds for the disabled. He was willing to walk to raise funds for others less well off – and he did it without damage to his feet!

Some of those men were lovely characters. They were able not only to help themselves and look after themselves, but wanted to help others also.

Not all the stories I could tell would be nearly as cheerful and successful. There was one elderly man – let's call him Mr Ba – who came in a very poor state, dirty and neglected, with far advanced leprosy. We discovered that because of his family's dread of catching the disease they had literally bricked him into a room of their flat in a high-rise block in Kowloon City. They fed him through a servery door. For years no-one ever touched him.

Eventually he was set free and brought over to us. We did what we could to clean him up but it was going to be a very long haul. His hands were very badly deformed, he had lost most of his toes, his face was deformed. We knew that eventually we could do some surgery, but first we had to control his leprosy. He'd had no treatment and so he was infectious on arrival.

However, he was soon non-infectious. That was the tragedy. His family had simply failed to understand that with treatment, even at home, he would not have given them leprosy. But they had walled him up – literally – with a disease which could readily have been treated, so that he need never have got those deformities.

With us he was better off than he had ever been. Nobody was afraid of him here. Everyone was trying to help themselves and him too. Lots of our patients worked as medical orderlies and taught him the exercises and helped him to oil and massage his hands and feet. Because of his poor general health he was admitted to the hospital, and slowly improved.

Then one night, (in the dim night light), he got up, slipped, and fell with a crunch, breaking his hip. That he had osteoporosis was not to be wondered at. Sitting in one room with a poor diet for ten years would not leave much calcium in the bones.

There was no way that we could get him admitted to a Hong Kong hospital, even though we had quite a good rapport with them and used to send other patients over for treatment. So I got out my old text books and read up ways of treating this sort of fractured hip. I found an article about erecting what was called "Arabian traction" – I do not know why it was called that – a method which was manageable, which would keep the leg in the required position and yet enable the staff to nurse and look after him while the hip healed. So we got him rigged up. He was not in pain and was doing quite well.

His relatives came on the boat on Sundays to visit him. One day when his wife was leaving, she asked the nurse, "Is he all right?" She replied that he was better than he was when he came in. "His broken hip will mend; there is nothing to worry about."

The wife responded, "He said he would be dead tomorrow night!" We looked at her amazed. I said, "We do not know of any particular reason why that should be unless he himself has decided that he wants to die." (Superstition is strong in Hong Kong.)

His wife returned to Hong Kong. On the Monday morning he was the same, no problems. That evening he did not want his dinner, but that was not too unusual with some patients. The nurse just settled him for the night. About midnight, the nurse rang to say he was dead.

We never discovered why. An autopsy did not reveal the cause. This is something which happens in Third World countries. I guess it happens in Australia too. He had literally decided that life was not worth living. He had a fractured hip, he had a disease which in his mind and in his family's mind was incurable. Although he had come to the only place in Hong Kong where he could really be looked after properly, he had decided to depart this life.

We had a number of patients who did the same sort of thing as Mr Ba.

9

Defeating Deformity – a Key Discovery

In 1959 it was widely believed that once you had leprosy you never 'came off the books' – you stayed on treatment for the rest of your life. If your feet had certain kinds of problems, the experts said that nothing could be done about it; they would just slowly get worse until the foot had to be amputated.

Because of these expectations, at that time the leprosy hospitals in India were packed full of life-long patients. But in Hong Kong there was a constant trickle of patients leaving the island. We needed that to happen to make room for more. We did not aim to be a long-term home. Only the affected person was admitted, not the whole family.

Some came as children. JayJay was fourteen when I first met him, and his leprosy was well controlled. His feet were not too bad; his hands were quite clawed but they weren't stiff, though he had already worn away part of some of his finger tips. So we put him on our rehabilitation surgery list. First I did the right hand, straightening the fingers, and later making the thumb move better so that he could pinch with the thumb against the finger tips. Then we did the left hand so that he now had two hands which looked good and were usable.

A year or so later he left us and went back to Hong Kong to his family where they apprenticed him to a carpenter. But JayJay had never really learnt to take care of himself properly. He had no major problems before he left us, although his finger tips had been shortened by the force he used whenever he gripped anything. He gripped things so hard he produced little blisters and wounds under the skin in his fingers, and when these had healed, his fingers were that little bit shorter than before. (We call it 'absorption' because the little bones at the end of the fingers are gradually absorbed or worn away by repetitive trauma.)

JayJay had not recognised the problem as it was happening, nor had we at that time. Although we attempted to teach patients to care for themselves, there is a very true maxim: "A person will only learn what is relevant to him at the time it is taught." JayJay did not appreciate that his hands had reduced pain perception. He did not try to care for them even though we had tried to teach him how. So when he went out he enjoyed his carpentry work, but failed to realise he was using such excessive strength in his grip.

Aged twenty, four years later, Jayjay came back and held out his hands. I do not think he had one finger that was of normal length – they were all short, stubby or bent, and he said, "I did not realise how strongly I was gripping my tools."

You can imagine a teenager learning to use chisels and hammers without pain's warning. He hammers a nail, hits his fingers and feels no pain. He damages his hand with a saw, or gets splinters in it. It gets infected but it does not hurt. JayJay had literally destroyed his hands while he was working. At that period in the sixties we were learning how vital it was to teach patients very carefully how to use their hands, wearing protective gloves if necessary, and the right sort of shoes. Although they may feel some touch, it is pain that is the protector. So we had to start a 'war' on patients destroying themselves. These problems are similar in diabetes and other diseases that affect nerves.

The problems of chronic nerve damage were, and still are, of great concern to us. In 1960 reconstructive surgery had not yet become a well accepted method of correcting deformity. It had been started in India in the early 1950s and TLM doctors had been doing it regularly in Hong Kong since 1958, but the lack of good physiotherapy for patients operated on initially meant disappointing results. After hand surgery some seemed to be no better off a couple of years later.

I eventually recognised the problem – the physiotherapy had been inadequate to train the patients to use their transferred tendons automatically in everyday use. Once back on their old job they resumed the old methods of work, especially in the way they gripped an object, and the transferred muscle eventually ceased to function. We say the muscle suffers from disuse atrophy, because it is not used enough to keep the fibres working adequately.

For many patients with severe loss of feeling, the only way they can be sure they are holding an object firmly is by gripping it so hard that the muscle, if it could, would yell in protest. For example, when driving a car a patient with severe damage to the nerve function in his hands will grip the wheel with maximum strength – that is the only way he knows that he has control over the wheel. If he drives for an hour he will hold it fiercely all the time. The strength of grip means that the blood in the finger tips cannot get through the little vessels and so some of the small cells die in that time, leading eventually to a shortening of the finger, as had happened to JayJay. A person with a normally sensitive hand would soon develop an ache, such as "writer's cramp", and would change to the other hand, or relax one hand to allow the blood to get through.

We realised that we needed to teach more occupational therapy – the correct way to do things – teaching it till it was automatic even when the patient was thinking about something else. It was years before I fully realised what I have been explaining above – why these patients were not gaining the maximum benefit from their surgery. When Jean Watson improved the whole physiotherapy program these problems diminished.

I had originally accepted the Hay Ling Chau job as a temporary position only; I had no intention of staying for long. The Chinese doctor whom I replaced did not return, so Doug Harman and I ran the institution till he went on leave to UK in mid-1960, expecting to return. I carried on, but I was not sure that I wanted his job permanently. I did not realise at that stage the potential that was to emanate from that appointment. The door was opening, but I could not see through the cracks. In those early days, I was asking myself, and God, "Why am I here?"

God knew why. He had to find a way to get me there and keep me there, and the way he chose was the tempting "carrot" of rehabilitation surgery, which had commenced in 1958, the year before I arrived. Here was my big chance – though originally I did not realise it. I had the ability and enough of the required training and experience to do the surgery. No-one in Hong Kong was bothered that I did not hold a higher surgical degree. In fact, once it became obvious that we were getting good results, I started to receive requests to operate on non-leprosy patients belonging to "fully trained and qualified surgeons" in Hong Kong.

The mission headquarters in London had another English doctor in the pipeline, Stuart Goodwin. En route he stopped off at Karigiri in South India to learn reconstructive surgery, and he did not arrive in Hong Kong until after Doug had left. By that time I was Acting Medical Superintendent, though still only a locum tenens, and it was expected that when my locum job ended I would leave Hong Kong.

It had become obvious however that a lone doctor could not cope with all the work waiting to be done there. The mission was very keen that I should become a full staff member and stay on, especially when in 1961 it became clear that Doug would not return. I was then offered the job as Medical Superintendent, and in 1962 I became a full member of the Mission to Lepers. (Its official name change to The Leprosy Mission (TLM) happened in 1966).

If I was going to do a good job I needed to learn more about surgery and its possibilities. Initially it was mostly tendon transfers. Each patient had to do his or her own physiotherapy to prepare for this surgery. This became better organised and more successful, after the arrival of Jean Watson.

Unless patients were able to improve the mobility and the suppleness of their skin, they were not good candidates for surgery, as they probably would not do enough exercises after surgery to get the transferred tendons working properly. So we chose the patients for whom there was a reasonable chance of getting a good result. It was essential that patients realised: yes, if you want deformities corrected, it can be done, *if* you do your share of the work. Good and lasting results would be important – especially as some of the early results had not lasted well.

In leprosy there are only a small number of nerves regularly affected, and these produce a predictable series of problems.

The 'foot-drop' is the most disabling – when the muscles on the front of the leg are no longer able to lift the front of the foot off the ground while the patient's heel is on the ground. This problem is similar to that experienced by many stroke victims. Foot-drop is often accompanied by clawed toes, when the toes bend up and the ball of the foot becomes more prominent as it hits the ground. Without corrective surgery, the toes often rub on the shoe, especially if the box of the shoe, the piece over the toes, is too low or too tight. This produces ulcers, but the patient is unaware of them, as they are painless.

In the hands, the nerves that are most commonly affected are the ones that run into the hand to make the small muscles in the hand function. When these muscles are paralysed a 'claw hand' like JayJay's results, in which the fingers tend to bend (flex) over at the little joints so that the patient is unable to straighten out the fingers, and the thumb is tucked back so that it is lying parallel to the palm of the hand and cannot be moved out to pinch. This type of hand gives a very poor grip. There is great difficulty in picking up objects, particularly round ones. The thumb cannot move out to grip a drinking glass or other cylindrical object. We can do a lot of things for these hands but most of them require several staged operations, so the patient undergoes two or three procedures at different times.

The face is another problem, being of course the first thing that attracts attention. In leprosy the nose is often deformed and damaged. There may also be paralysis of the muscles of the lower half of the face. Some patients lose their eyebrows. They may also have big, loose baggy ears, which they would like trimmed. These are relatively minor things, were it not for the cosmetic and the stigma factor.

The crucial facial disability of leprosy is inability to shut the eyelids, which need to close to prevent ulcers on the eye that could destroy vision. Surgery to the eyelids is one of the few facial operations that we will strongly encourage the patient to have. A patient may not realise how dangerous it is to be unable to blink away an irritation. Although we only operate if the person is willing, and while for many of the deformities some patients will say, "It does not matter, I can manage", we cannot allow a leprosy patient to lose his sight when he has already lost sensation in his hands and feet.

All these disabilities and the scope for their surgical correction were well known by the time I came into leprosy – but there was another aspect that soon had me very involved.

In early 1960 I was confronted in the outpatient ulcer clinic by a young man, Chung, whose foot was very swollen. It was not painful – there was nothing wrong with it, as far as he was concerned – it was just swollen and a bit warm and had been like that for maybe a couple of months. So I sent him in for an X-ray.

We had our own X-ray equipment. A routine was already established that every patient, on arrival, had baseline X-rays taken of chest, hands and feet. These were repeated every year to record progress. A baseline X-ray is excellent for dealing with people who have nerve damage in their hands and feet because it lets you see the state of the bones on first encounter. If, at a future date, a patient such as Chung has a hot swollen foot, a new X-ray will show if there is any fracture.

Chung's new X-ray showed that he had a new fracture in one of the bones near his ankle (the navicular bone). I took the X-ray in to Dr Harman and said, "Chung has this fracture in his navicular; will I put it in a plaster?" (This was the usual treatment.) Doug looked at the X-ray and said "Oh, yes, he's obviously fractured it. But it is no use putting it into plaster – these fractures will never heal."

I asked, "Why do not they?"

"Oh, we do not know why, but you read the books – they all tell you that the fractures in a foot with nerve damage will not heal. If you treat them in a plaster cast, after a while they appear on X-ray to be getting better, but as soon as you take the cast off, they break down again."

"Do you mind if I use a plaster?" I asked.

"No," he replied, "By all means, go ahead and do it." So I did. In the X-ray three months later, it looked as though the fracture was healing. I was very pleased with myself. It looked good enough to take the cast off and let him walk without it, and that is what I did. I repeated the X-rays at three months out of plaster to see what was happening. It looked as if the fracture was healed, but when I repeated the X-rays at six months out of the plaster, I realised that the affected bone and the adjacent bones were altering their shape. Subtle changes must have been happening all along without my recognising them.

Why did this happen? When the fracture had occurred, Chung's foot had become hot, which indicated that there was far more blood in the area than normal. This is called "hyperaemia" – literally increased blood supply, when the blood comes to help heal the bones. This is the natural healing process of bones. This increased blood supply removes calcium ready for the new bone structure to be laid down, and then the calcium returns. The calcium is removed from all the bones around the fracture site, so that they *all* become softer, not just the bone where the fracture has occurred.

What had happened to Chung was that, when the foot looked good on X-ray, it showed that the bones were uniting, but the calcium had not yet returned. So when he started to walk, the pressure of walking was little by little changing the shape of the softened bones, even though they looked as if they were healed. With normal pain perception he would have protected the foot because it would have "hurt" – but no pain, no self-protection. Hence his walking was slowly pushing the bones out of shape. Over the next six months they changed more. The fracture itself was still intact. It was healed; the bones had not broken again – but he had this subtle deformity of his foot that he would keep for the rest of his life.

I did not know what to do about it. The books that I had gave no suggestions; they just said the bones would not heal. The type of deformity that could develop was said to be a Charcot foot, named after the French neurologist who first described the problem. The fact that healing had not been regularly observed led to the conviction that no healing was possible for these bone problems. Therefore many orthopaedic surgeons said it was not worth treating a Charcot foot.

I decided just to continue watching and waiting. The next X-ray – nine months after the cast came off – showed that the bones were now far better calcified and there had been no further change in the shape since the one at six months.

It was also obvious that the foot no longer got warm when the patient was walking – no increased blood supply. So this set me thinking: is this the reason why people said that these fractures did not heal? The fracture I had treated was only a small one; we had got it healed and it had remained healed. But the weakness of the bones, which was partly a natural response to the fracture and to healing, had encouraged deformity of the adjacent bones when walking was resumed without the cast, because there was no pain to warn the patient that he was damaging himself. One could reason that if the foot had had a major fracture, then we probably wouldn't have been so fortunate. Chung had only had a minor fracture.

But with some fractures, the pieces of broken bone are pulled quite a distance apart. So even if they were to heal, they wouldn't be firm – certainly not in the few weeks that would normally be the time in plaster for a foot with normal pain sensation. With normal sensation the patient would not put his full weight on it as it would be too painful. But Chung had not had that advantage. We were able to learn so much from that one patient because of good examinations, X-rays and record keeping.

Over the years that followed, I came to realise that if one is treating a fracture in any foot in which there is reduced pain sensation, one needs to keep the cast on two to three times longer than for the same fracture in a normal foot which feels pain. As far as we could tell – and we checked this with pathology biopsies in later years – the bone healing was normal, but leprosy patients put so much stress on the healing bones when a walking cast is removed that they break down whatever healing has taken place. This was why the books said "such fractures will not heal." The many series of X-rays showed how a patient's foot would completely break down and become useless – so grossly at times that it required amputation – if a small fracture remained untreated, even though detected.

We decided not to use the term "Charcot" to describe a foot deformed by these tragically neglected fractures. That term conveyed to most doctors that healing would never occur. In later years my associates and I used the term Neuropathic Bone Disorganisation, or disintegration (NBD).

Amputation is often adopted as the easy solution to the problem of an infected or deformed foot. For a patient who cannot feel pain however, it produces other, very different problems that may be even more difficult to deal with.

There was one big man, Ah Tung, who had fractured one of his ankle bones but who also had been allowed to keep walking. Eventually, the main leg bone, the tibia, went right through the heel bone and he ended up walking on the tibia, with a huge ulcer over it. Eventually he had his leg amputated; this all happened before I arrived. That may have solved the problem of the deformity and the ulceration of his foot, but getting an artificial leg to fit that stump, which lacked normal sensation, was much more difficult than finding a shoe to fit an oddly shaped foot. Finally a dedicated prosthesis maker was able to find a way to help him, but only after immense trouble, trial and error.

We found quite a number of patients with similar problems to Chung's. I would put them in plaster casts and keep them in casts for many months. Most feet we saved – far better to have long-term plaster casts if it could save a foot. An amputation is for ever. It did not take us long before we had 'follow-ups' of patients – six, twelve months, two years after a fracture had healed. Chung's later X-rays showed that the fracture site was firm and that further deformity had not occurred after the removal of the cast. Hence by "accident" – another of these God-directed happenings – I had stumbled onto a treatment principle that has changed the whole outlook in the treatment of many patients with problem painless feet. These feet **will** heal if protected in a cast for long enough.

Paul Brand had shown that ulcers stated to be non-healing would heal in plaster casts. We were on the threshold of showing that the dreaded disintegrating bones of neuropathic feet would also heal if placed in a suitable plaster cast for an extra length of time. This would prevent hundreds of amputations. This principle is the basis for much of the work I now do with many non-leprosy patients in Australia (like Daren in the opening chapter), and those with similar problems who keep arriving at my clinics, in Australia and elsewhere.

So much for Chung! A couple of years later, his foot was still satisfactory. There was some deformity, but he could wear a normal shoe, provided that the shoe had a good protective insole and that he wore a good pair of socks. I am quite sure that if we had not put it in that plaster cast at that stage, he would have ended up with a severely deformed foot. I saw lots of patients later with such badly deformed feet.

10

Spreading the word – early outreach

Early in 1960 an American surgeon, who was working in Taiwan, visited us to see what we were doing. He asked if it would be possible for one of us to go to Taiwan and suggest ways of improving their leprosy program. Doug Harman was going to UK in June and so we decided that I could take my holidays and go to Taiwan in May. By this time I was quite capable of doing the basic surgery and of assessing who would benefit from the surgery.

In May 1960 I flew into Taipei, where everyone pulled together to make my trip memorable. I was to travel round the island clockwise, starting with Whalien on the north-east coast. Here I stayed with the German Sisters who ran the leprosy program.

I next visited Pingdung, then Tainan where I stayed with Ruth Lin. An American nurse, she had worked in China till missionaries had to leave, and was then running leprosy programs in Taiwan. She had married a Chinese, Frank Lin, and they founded the *Lin An* Church in Tainan. A quick flight took me across to Makung on the Pescadores Islands where Marjorie Bly, also an ex-China American nurse, ran the leprosy program based in the local provincial hospital. Next I visited Chungwha Christian Hospital and the outpatient clinic run by Gerda Beck and Sister (Dr) Antonio Maria, before heading back to Taipei to see the leprosy program in the Mackay Hospital, and finally the Lo Sheng Government Leprosy Hospital on the outskirts of Taipei.

It was a fascinating trip. I found a chain of well organised clinics run by nurses. Most had no doctor, or if one was involved he probably knew little about leprosy, so the nurses solved their own problems. I taught some simple physiotherapy en route – this was something that had not yet been started and was certainly needed – and there were a lot of deformities that could relatively easily be corrected by the right surgery. Not only did I see the deformities of leprosy but many deformities from poliomyelitis epidemics. A person with a foot-drop was assumed to have had polio – so polio reduced the problem of leprosy stigma.

I could see much that needed to be done. There were capable nurses who needed a doctor who understood and could realistically deal with the specific problems of leprosy.

Here God gave me a vision. There was a real need for someone who could travel round the various centres here in Taiwan and I assumed – rightly – in many other centres in the world to teach and solve the problems on the spot, considering the various social and cultural needs. When I joined the mission a year or two later, it was with the proviso that I would be able to travel and teach as conditions allowed. God used that visit to Taiwan to sow the seeds that would mature into my future extensive "Wanderings".

Soon after my return to Hong Kong we said farewell to Dr Doug Harman and his wife Gladys, off to UK for leave. It was accepted that I, then the Medical Officer-in-Charge, would remain in that position until he returned.

The next important visitor was Dr Christopher Maddox, another senior China veteran with the Overseas Missionary Fellowship (OMF was the new name of the China Inland Mission). In 1952 he had founded the Christian hospital at Manorom in central Thailand. Chris came to Hong Kong for "rest" to recover from illness. He came across to see what we were doing, because leprosy was a developing part of the Manorom Hospital program. He scrubbed in with me for a hand operation and was fascinated at the possibilities it offered his own patients. He asked if Manorom's Dr June Morgan could come over to work with me to learn. We scheduled that for early 1961. When June came we did a lot of surgery in order to teach her the techniques. She learnt a number of operations and much physiotherapy and other aspects of leprosy care. I think we changed her whole attitude to leprosy and its management.

As a follow-up to their visits, in January 1962 I made my way to Thailand. Manorom Hospital was then a six hour bus trip from Bangkok. It was very cold and the wind literally whistled through the canvas sides of the bus. I was even glad to be able buy hot coffee served in an old condensed milk tin! Thailand has come a long way since then.

At the hospital, my schedule had been organised so that I would be there for the opening of the new leprosy wing, built to accommodate the patients, with their outpatient clinics, physiotherapy and handcrafts. The day I arrived we selected a patient for surgery – a middle-aged man with far advanced leprosy. He had ulcerated feet, badly destroyed hands and a collapsed nose. The first job was to clean him up ready for surgery, so I spent hours doing all that. No one had ever done that for him before. Culturally the Thai would not expect anyone to handle their feet in that way. He was a quick learner and soon learnt to soak and treat his feet and hands himself. He soon realised how much better and how much more comfortable his feet were. Although they lack pain perception, even so-called anaesthetic feet do have some sort of sensation.

From then on he would turn up at clinics and tell the other patients how good it was to look after themselves well. This teaching coming from a patient was far more effective than from a staff member. Patients could not say to him, "You do not know what it is like to live with feet that do not feel properly."

I went out with the nurses to outpatient clinics, riding pushbikes down sand tracks by the river. I had not ridden a bike for ages – but I managed! This gave me a glimpse into the world in which these patients have to survive, and in which the missionary nurses were seeking to help them: open fires, metal cooking pots, candles or kerosene lamps, bare wooden floors – and footwear taken off at the door. All houses are up steps, as large areas flood each year. No wonder there were many burns on hands and splinters in feet!

I spent about ten days at Manorom; we did a number of operations and taught the nurses – mostly Westerners – a lot about leprosy. Then I took the night train north to Chiang Mai where I visited the McKean Institute for the first time. I made many trips to McKean over the next 40 years. In 1962 some rehabilitation had commenced, but very little was happening. The patients did their own physio with little teaching or assistance, and, looking back, I wonder how effective it was. The hospital was basically a collection of many small cottages where leprosy patients lived and expected to live for the rest of their lives. There were wards for those sick enough to need extra care, but little or no reconstructive surgery. The institute was run by the Church of Christ in Thailand, and efforts were being made to update its work to bring it in line with the newer concepts that Dr Brand taught. Over the next ten years there would be an influx of expatriate staff to teach and do various forms of rehabilitation and occupational therapy. On that visit I was just a tourist with an unusual interest in leprosy.

Meanwhile the work in Hong Kong was going to plan. Dr Stuart Goodwin had settled in and was doing regular clinics and surgery. The medical students came out in groups, about once a month. Various visitors came to see what we were doing and this included some Hong Kong surgeons interested in the operations, which were not those they had learnt. Some of them were interested in learning these operations for their private patients. I could never be sure how well these observers really learned. Some certainly did not!

Doctors, nurses and physiotherapists came from other countries to observe and learn from us. I could see that there were unlimited possibilities to help improve the quality of care in many centres. The fact that we were actively trying to rehabilitate patients was not lost on the world at large. I was invited to do a presentation at the Pan Pacific Conference for the Rehabilitation of the Disabled to be held in Manila in November 1962. That would be my first big international conference. That was followed by a trip to India as told in chapter 11, and three months' work in Thailand, in 1963. Over the next few years I made trips to Papua-New Guinea, Japan, Korea, Malaya and Singapore which are dealt with in other chapters.

In 1966-7 TLM was asked if someone could be sent to Pakistan to assist in upgrading a leprosy program. Because of the political situation they asked me to go instead of trying to send an experienced Indian.

The government owned and ran the so-called "Leprosy Home" at Manghopir. It was a typical "home" with minimal facilities which the German Christustrager Mission was upgrading, providing proper hospital facilities. They had also brought in a doctor and nurses to improve care. In the previous decade Dr Ruth Pfau (associated with the Marie Adelaide Leprosy Centre (MALC) in Karachi) and Dr Zarina Fazelbhoy (a Pakistani dermatologist) had set up a simple roadside "clinic" outside the gate, to provide medical essentials for the leprosy sufferers.

Pakistan is an endemic leprosy area. The estimate of numbers of patients in Pakistan has varied enormously. At one stage I think they said there were 200,000, but that figure was cut back when they discovered that many of the patients were registered at two or three different clinics.

On that first visit I lived with the German staff at Nizimabad and worked at Manghopir most of the time. I was confronted with many deformities, some very severe and often grossly neglected. None of the patients were really prepared for surgery. We assessed them and started doing physiotherapy. I worked with the German shoe makers to improve the quality and versatility of their footwear. When the operation room was functional we were able to do the first operations in the new centre. I had to select carefully because the post-operative physiotherapy had to be left to one of the nurses, Sister Gisela, who although she had never done it before, became very efficient.

All water had to be brought in by tanker. The first patient literally walked into the operation room – we had to start by washing the sand off his feet! Sand was everywhere; Manghopir was on the edge of the desert. Nevertheless the first few operations were highly successful, so patients were encouraged to exercise to prepare for the next time surgery was available, and live in hope that their turn would come. We gave one man a new set of eyebrows and such procedures became really popular.

There was a young physician just out of Germany, so I spent a good deal of time with him on the medical aspects of care. In that high temperature and low humidity one of the big problems was dehydration. Many high fevers would settle rapidly when patients drank enough water. We made sure they drank plenty by giving each patient a clay water pot by the bed, filled four times daily. They had to have their pot empty by the time the water carrier next came around!! Most of the fevers vanished in a few days.

I returned there in 1969 and stayed with the German sisters, now living in a house in the hospital grounds. Again I worked mainly at Manghopir, but started going to the MALC, and also to the Spencer Eye Hospital in Karachi. But I had a new friend to make. Sister Adelheide Nestle had just arrived from Germany in response to a message from Sister Gisela that a trained physiotherapist was needed. Adelheide had originally trained as a nurse, then as a physiotherapist. A lovely girl, extremely capable – and I was able to be her teacher.

Once she understood what was needed, she found patients when I was not there and prepared them for surgery, determining what they were able to cope with. Adelheide could train others to be physiotherapy assistants. Then when I arrived, she would take over as supervisor in the operating room, overseeing the local assistants in doing all the sterilising and preparation needed. I was thrilled when in 2005 she received Pakistani government recognition for her humanitarian service.

It was about this time that I met Dr Gool Talati. She was a plastic surgeon, trained in UK and was now back in Karachi and prepared to help. She did beautiful surgery and soon learnt our economical methods of providing anaesthesia and selecting those who really wanted to help themselves. She was an expert on face and nose reconstruction and taught me much. We shared an interest in hands, but I had to share with her the best methods of doing tendon transfers in feet. She became the mainstay of the reconstructive program for the next couple of decades, working solidly between my trips.

In February 1971 I was again in Pakistan for the one and only All Pakistan Leprosy Conference. We had doctors from East Pakistan, just before it separated and became Bangladesh. Dr Stanley Browne and I were there and we stayed as the house guests of Dr Zarina Fazelbhoy and her husband Akbar. Even as we were leaving Karachi at the end of February there was a lot of unrest leading to the breakaway. In the car en route to the airport to fly out, my host stated he was glad we were leaving as he did not know if he could ensure our safety in the weeks ahead, given the situation that was blowing up.

In 1973 during a short stop-over in Karachi en route to Bergen (Chapter 16), I first met Dr Thomas Chiang who had just started to work at the MALC as the junior doctor. Much of the future acceptance and prestige of the MALC would depend on Thomas. He was rapidly learning the craft of caring for leprosy. He was a lovely Christian man, a member of the Roman Catholic church, born and trained in Dhaka when it was East Pakistan. He had not long qualified from medical school when the split came and East Pakistan became Bangladesh.

With thousands of others, Thomas migrated to Pakistan while he could. So he was officially a Pakistani citizen – and he was Chinese and a Roman Catholic! This made him very different in his attitudes to the patients and their problems from the usual medical appointee one encountered in Karachi. Thomas brought with him the skills, the ability and the concern for patients that I had become used to when working with the Chinese people. He was a very keen student of all that I was doing, and on my future visits he was soon learning from me to do reconstructive surgery, although he had had no formal surgical training. Well, nor had I, so I understood that and appreciated his efforts to learn.

In the mid-seventies the Pakistan government took over Manghopir and ran it themselves, gradually phasing out the German staff. This certainly meant that the standards of some of the work also fell – but Dr Gool and I were able to continue to operate and help in many ways until the mid-eighties.

11

India, Paul Brand – and more travels

In 1962 we established a working system in Hong Kong. Dr Stuart Goodwin had arrived in 1961 from UK. We shared the general medical clinics in the mornings. As there was a lot of surgery to be done, we then both spent afternoons operating, sometimes together, sometimes separately. Jean Watson came to share my house and our paths would be intertwined professionally for many years ahead.

I had been appointed the Medical Superintendent of Hay Ling Chau and Alan Waudby was Administrative Superintendent. Now we could plan for the future. With surgery one of my main interests, it was decided that I should go to work with Dr Paul Brand in Vellore/Karigiri in India, while Stuart Goodwin was available to run Hay Ling Chau. Paul Brand, originally from England, was already by this time becoming well-known in world Christian mission and medical circles for his work among leprosy patients. His story has been told in several excellent books, first in *Ten Fingers for God* by Dorothy Clarke Wilson and later in *The Gift of Pain* co-written with Philip Yancey. With Philip, Paul also wrote *Fearfully and Wonderfully Made* and *In His Image.* These made him widely known and admired. His career, later based in America, continued to be distinguished over the years. We all mourned his loss at his death in 2004. The world had lost a marvellous man.

In late 1962 I attended the Pan Pacific Conference for the Rehabilitation of the Disabled held in Manila. Then I spent a week's holiday amid village life in nearby Calapan on Mindoro Island, where I did a bit of medical work. I then returned briefly to Hong Kong before leaving just after Christmas for India via Singapore.

This was the first of many visits to Singapore and I stayed for a day or two at the OMF headquarters. It was dark when the taxi pulled up at the door. I rang the bell and the door was opened by an Australian about ten years my senior. I said "Are you expecting Dr Warren?" The answer: "Oh, yes". "Well, I am Dr Warren." He looked rather startled, picked up my bag, walked up the stairs and showed me to a room. I found out later that the reason he was so taken aback was that he'd heard about a doctor who was teaching at the hospital at Manorom in Central Thailand and who was friends with Dr Chris Maddox (probably the most senior of the OMF doctors at that time). He somehow expected someone Dr Maddox's age – a grey-haired old lady! No wonder he was surprised – I was only 33 at the time! Anyway we had a good laugh and became good friends. I flew on to Colombo, then to Madras and then went by train to Karigiri where Paul Brand met me. He had arranged for me to stay with an Indian family about forty minutes' walk from the hospital.

For the next eight weeks I worked at Vellore, the main hospital, or at Karigiri, the specialised Leprosy Unit. Clinics, ward rounds, discussion groups and operating room sessions followed. I especially appreciated a series of lectures that Paul presented on the surgery of the hand; I still have those notes today. Quite often at lunch Paul and I would meet in the canteen and discuss patients we had seen. I enjoyed these sessions because Paul, in spite of his many years on the job, treated me as an equal and was quite prepared to discuss the pros and cons of some method I had learnt or developed that was not the same as the one he used. Considering I had only been doing this surgery for less than four years, and had had no official training, it was very gracious of him and it became obvious that he appreciated how much I had learnt already.

I went to the Schieffelin Leprosy Research and Training Centre at Karigiri in the hospital bus. It was a residential hospital where patients often stayed for many months while a series of operations were carried out. Students from all over Asia stayed there learning how to care for those with leprosy.

At Karigiri I became more familiar with "*Charcot foot*" – the dreaded bone disintegration that in Hong Kong I was already treating by plaster casting, with good results. The Karigiri staff followed the standard text books, accepting that a Charcot joint or bone problem would not heal. But I had been finding otherwise. Did my experience and experiments alter their ideas? I may never know. Certainly my techniques did not become routine there for many years.

There were many points in medical management, even in those days, in which my routines differed from those used by the staff at Karigiri. I tried to share these and my efforts often resulted in worthwhile discussions. A major factor was that there are definite racial variations in the complications that develop in leprosy. The Indians did not get nearly as many severe complications as I had had to deal with in Chinese sufferers like poor Mr Ba (see Chapter 8). I had a lot to share with them about the most serious lepra reactions, which are common in the lighter skinned races, but relatively rare in the darker skinned Indians.

There were three doctors from Thailand among the students there at the same time. I did not realise at that time what a "coincidence" this was, and what a helpful effect it would have on my later acceptance into the Thai medical fraternity. How do you define coincidence? I say, "A co-incidence is two happenings that God brings together for his purposes." Because of that brief period studying together those men accepted me as if I had gone to the same medical college, and this in Thailand brings all sorts of benefits. It made me readily acceptable as a consultant when I started visiting Thailand regularly.

I was in and out of Paul and Margaret Brand's house which was close to mine. I got to know their children, and enjoyed being part of their family. Margaret told me about the first time she went to the

UK with a couple of small children, by boat as was usual in those days. On arrival at the docks in the UK the customs officer was being very fussy and had just finished emptying the first box and pointed to the second. "What is in there?" Margaret said: "Those are my children's toys and presents that the leprosy patients have given us to bring home." "Oh!" said the man, as a look of fear raced across his face. He then ticked the box and all the other boxes and let them go.

I never forgot that. For years when I packed to go through airports I made sure that my teaching materials were on top of my suitcase, easily seen as soon as the case was opened. The poster "Leprosy can be cured" was a good one, or the book *Leprosy for Paramedical Workers* – and I would drape a stethoscope across the top. Many customs officers were so afraid of leprosy they would not dig into the case, fearing it might be contaminated. One of the few times and places where the fear of leprosy is an advantage!

Paul was the surgeon who realised that much could be done to reconstruct hands deformed by leprosy. He had come to the Vellore Christian Hospital in about 1946, when they urgently needed a surgeon in order to have properly qualified staff for registration as an accredited medical college. He went to India within the first decade of the use of dapsone as an effective drug for treating leprosy. Early in his time in India he was confronted with the deformities of leprosy and challenged with, "Now that we have a drug to treat leprosy, why do the patients still get deformity? And why is the deformity not cured by dapsone?" No one knew. No one really knew why leprosy patients' limbs became deformed.

Paul gathered some keen doctors around him and set to work to find out. The story is wonderfully told in the book *Ten Fingers for God* by Dorothy Clarke Wilson. By the time I got to India he had found out that leprosy affects nerves and destroys their ability to carry messages. This results in muscles that will not move and skin that does not feel heat or pain. As a result the patients damage themselves and then go on using the damaged limb, preventing healing. Paul showed that nerve damage was the reason why many of their problems developed. He recognised that the main deformities of most leprosy patients could be corrected by half a dozen operations. Some of these operations were those used for other diseases, but he modified some and invented others that are now being used by doctors round the world for treating similar problems in non-leprosy patients. Tendon transplants in hands, feet, and faces could greatly enhance the social acceptance and ability of the patient.

His wife, Margaret, was also a doctor, initially without speciality training. In India she realised that leprosy patients had many eye problems and very little was being done to help prevent the patients going blind. She took up this challenge and became an internationally recognised eye specialist for leprosy patients.

During my eight weeks I also visited a number of other leprosy centres in South India. When I finished at Vellore, I travelled across India to Bombay to spend a short time with Dr Antia, a plastic surgeon who was doing reconstructive procedures for leprosy patients and others. From there I went to Calcutta in order to obtain a visa into Thailand, but finding I had to wait a week for it, I went to Darjeeling in the Himalayas, popular as a cooler summer retreat. The headmaster of the school there was Dave Stewart, a university friend of my brother, whom I also had known at Sydney University.

I had been asked to do a locum at the Christian hospital at Manorom in Thailand, where I had visited in 1962. Dr June Morgan was in the UK on leave and I was asked me to go back to run the leprosy program while she was away – hence the need for the Thai visa.

I stayed at the OMF guest house in Bangkok. The hostess asked me to see Gopa, a young woman from a well-to-do family with obviously deformed hands and an ulcerated deformed foot. I arranged for her to come to Manorom with me – in fact it was very convenient as she met me at the railway station and actually took me there! I spoke no Thai of course and hardly knew my way around.

At Manorom I worked at the OMF hospital and in the outpatient leprosy clinics scattered around the countryside, teaching the staff how to look after leprosy patients. I also assisted in other branches of medicine, especially obstetrics, general surgery and trauma. I was able to operate on Gopa and improve the appearance and function of her hands and her problem foot. During her time at Manorom she became a Christian. Her whole life was transformed. She later did a bible training course and worked as an evangelist, a "Bible woman". She still keeps contact with me, meeting me and entertaining me to a meal when I have time while visiting Thailand.

I had a fascinating time teaching some of the other doctors reconstructive surgery. One day I was asked by the dentist to see a girl in her late teens who, when very young, had had a bad fall, breaking the jaw joint beside her left ear. The bones had fused together and she could not open her mouth. She had to live on soft food and fluids. I had never done the operation but – was it another of God's coincidences? – while in Vellore I had been in the operation room when a fellow Australian surgeon was operating to correct a similar problem. I was not actually assisting in the surgery, but one of God's gifts to me is that if I can see something being done, I can usually repeat it myself. So we looked it up in the books and I did it together with the dentist. The girl was thrilled that she could eat watermelon next day! Over the next month we did two more very similar operations. It was interesting that these three arrived within a month and yet there were no other patients needing that procedure before or since! Strange but true.

I spent 11 weeks at Manorom on that visit. I had expected to stay longer, but the Thai government declined to renew my visa – and this meant leaving in a hurry! I had just got to my seat on the plane when I heard the Thai hostess calling for "Mor Garuna!" "Mor" is the Thai word for doctor and "Garuna" is the Thai translation of "grace", so this was my Thai name. I sheepishly went up to check and found that Gopa's mother had arranged for a gift of Thai silk. Of course she did not know my English name – so it was just as well I had learnt a few Thai words!

So it was back to Hong Kong, to repack and wait for the boat to take me to Australia on leave. Missionaries' home leave, then called "furlough", was scarcely a holiday. All the deputation work, speaking at meetings etc, was really harder work for me than doing the regular medical work in Hong Kong. Today most missions call it home assignment or home service – a more accurate label.

Dr Goodwin had been in charge of the medical work in Hong Kong for almost six months. Alan Waudby looked after administration, and the two Chinese doctors could do a lot of the routine clinical and clerical work. Jean Watson had now set up the physiotherapy program and was training patients to be able to do the general day to day running of the program. It was a good time to leave, and I was able to obtain a berth on a cargo ship carrying only 12 passengers, going via North Borneo to Sydney. That trip took four weeks and was really relaxing. I could read and sew, knit and talk – no patients, no teaching, no deputation work!

At home, once I had acquired a car, the regular routine began of taking meetings and driving around, meeting people and raising funds. I drove many miles in the next six months and spoke at dozens of meetings. For some years I had been writing a circular letter, *Warren's Wanderings,* a few times a year to be sent out to my friends and TLM supporters. Now I had a chance to meet some of them and to increase my range of friends and acquaintances. More than once a well-educated white Australian refused to shake my hand for fear I might be carrying leprosy! Leprosy still (some 40 years later) evokes fear, not only in endemic areas, but here in

Australia, where it is rare.

A highlight of my time at home was a visit to Australia by Paul Brand. He had many meetings scheduled and, on 23rd December 1963, I had the privilege of driving him over 100 miles in the pre-Christmas traffic! So we had plenty of time to talk. We even managed to get him a visa to stop over in Thailand so he could visit some of his ex-students.

Paul knew of my affinity for reconstructive surgery and of course he also knew the Third World's needs. The usual route to becoming a surgeon was to do a traditional course of study and experience. He said: "You can already do most of the operations that your patients will need. You could go back to surgery school and study for four years, and you will learn a lot of things you will never use in leprosy, but may well learn very few things really needed to help leprosy patients. Without that extra degree you are acceptable in the Third World because you can do the work and you're willing to work with others." But he did advise me to give the entrance exam a go. He said, "Try it, but let's just leave the matter in God's hands – if you do not get through, just go and get on with the job and we will see what God has in store for you."

So from January 1964, I lived at the YWCA in Melbourne, attending lectures and practical work at the nearby Royal Australasian College of Surgeons. The exams? No, I did not pass. Yet, because of my experience in Hong Kong, I was teaching some of the other students the anatomy of the hand and forearm, which we had to know for the exams – but they had had no experience in that field.

So that was that. The next move came from the mission. They had been challenged with the needs of the leprosy work in New Guinea where very little had been done up to this point. Although there were clinics, TLM was hopeful of developing a rehabilitation program in New Guinea and already had people training in India.

But they needed centres for doing the surgery. True, there were government hospitals, mostly on the coast, but when New Guinea tribes-people leave their own tribal territory, they are in danger of being killed for trespassing. In New Guinea it was advisable to send the doctor to the patient, not the patient to the doctor. So TLM wanted advice as to where to set up small hospitals where the surgery could be done in the patients' own tribal areas.

I had visited the capital Port Moresby in 1961 en route between Hong Kong and Sydney, and had done some teaching. So I was obviously the one for the job. The eastern half of the large island of New Guinea was under Australian protection, so Australia was virtually responsible for the medical work though nationals were being trained. Also there were dozens, if not hundreds, of separate language groups in Papua- New Guinea; linguists were trying to record and write these languages so that tribes would have some of the Scriptures in their own language and not just the trade language, then called Pidgin, which was often inadequate for conveying bible truths.

I spent about six weeks travelling round the various centres, from the big coastal government hospitals up to smaller mission ones in the highlands. The doctor in charge of one hospital sported a splendid moustache and the locals called him "Dr Mouthgrass"! I ran a seminar on leprosy at a government hospital, demonstrating typical lesions and deformities. In thanks I was presented with a traditional Mount Hagen axe – a beautiful artefact I still have.

One of the last centres that I visited was the hospital at Balimo. This was run by the Unevangelised Fields Mission and I knew some of the staff. I was to fly from the highlands down to Balimo on a river delta on the coast. I was told that the Missionary Aviation Fellowship (MAF) plane would leave at dawn. We climbed into the little plane while it was still dark and taxied down the strip, which was no more than car tracks. As we took off, dawn broke around the tops of the surrounding mountains. There followed a most beautiful sunrise, which I will never forget. We were right in it – surrounded by pink-tipped and silver-edged clouds that seemed to cover the whole sky.

The hospital at Balimo had been established for a long time and was well set up. It provided medical facilities for a large area of the Fly River District and they also had outreach hospitals up in the hills. After assessing Balimo, I went back to Port Moresby and was able to operate at the local government hospital on patients from Gemo Island, the leprosy residential island. I performed surgery on two patients with foot-drop and one with a hand problem. I carefully instructed the nurses at Gemo on how to do the follow-up physiotherapy and was later told that the results for those three patients were all excellent. It certainly made a difference to the whole program, because, when the other patients in New Guinea saw the results on these three, they realised that we could do something. Now more patients were keen to do their exercises. So by the time Dr Ken Clezy, an Australian surgeon, came back late in 1964 from training in India, there was a queue of patients, ready, willing and just waiting to be told when they could have their surgery.

Ken was an excellent person for that job. He was quick and capable and he could teach others well. He would fly into the smaller centres, spend a few days operating and then go off, and the physiotherapist would come in later and get the patients using their transferred tendons. He really did far more leprosy surgical procedures per year, I think, than I ever did. So for a couple of years he was kept very busy in New Guinea till he had worked through the backlog, and then the work-load slackened off. He was still doing the surgery there until the end of the 1970s.

But when I returned to New Guinea in 1998, it was obvious that the standards of care which we had instituted in those days had not been maintained. In some areas no one even seemed to be able to diagnose leprosy, and, for those who had deformities, very little was being offered in the way of rehabilitation or physiotherapy, certainly at the centres that I visited.

At the end of my New Guinea trip I returned to Sydney and wrote a report for the mission. Mr McKeown, who was then TLM Australian Secretary, came to Sydney to discuss it with me before I flew back to Asia, via a rather circuitous route, but one that was going to bring many advantages.

12

Visitors and Unexpected Bonuses

In the mid-60s a significant visitor to Hay Ling Chau was George Bedbrook (later Sir George), who had a worldwide reputation for the work he had done in rehabilitation of the disabled in Perth, Western Australia. I showed him what we were doing in reconstructive surgery, special footwear and physiotherapy. Then we turned to the X-rays, especially of feet. I showed him sets like those of Chung, whose feet had remained functional and useful, even if one foot was somewhat deformed. I had dozens of examples of feet with similar deformities, feet with some abnormality of the bones considered untreatable. But as with Chung, I had found in many that with "rest and protect", healing could occur.

Before going to Australia on leave in 1963 I had seen a young man, Leung, with a chronically infected foot, in hospital on strict bed rest for many months. The ulcer was healing and I realized that he could soon start walking. I warned the staff that he should undertake a program of slowly increasing periods of walking and non-weight-bearing exercise, to encourage his bones to recalcify and so become strong.

A year later on my return to Hong Kong I saw Leung again. The foot was now ulcer free but abnormal in shape. New X-rays confirmed this. Against my advice he had been allowed to leave hospital early with no restriction on his walking. The foot became warm and swollen. As it was not painful he just kept walking while the foot slowly changed shape and the arch collapsed. It was certainly an odd shape, but as he could walk, he did not worry. The X-ray now showed that he had had a fracture that had healed in an abnormal position. Now if he kept walking on that foot he would get more ulcers, and would eventually lose the foot. The bones had recalcified; the foot now was not hot so there was no clinical reason to put him back in plaster, but I was very strict with his footwear to prevent more ulcers.

I showed his X-rays and called Leung to see Dr Bedbrook. He was very interested and helpful and carefully examined Leung, noting that the nerve did not function correctly. He knew Leung's problem was similar to others he had treated with nerve damage in their feet.

"Oh," he said, "you need to operate on that foot. Do an arthrodesis." I could find no reference to this in text books – they usually said nothing could be done – Dr Bedbrook explained what he meant and I did it and achieved a better shape. We, including Leung, were well satisfied with the foot's changed shape. But he spent almost a year in plaster casts before graduating to using correct shoes, and never going barefoot.

By then I had done similar operations for a number of other patients, with good results. I realized how I could diagnose these bone problems before they actually caused deformity, and how we could get the bones to heal in a functional position even after the deformity began to develop. None of this was in the text books, and certainly not in the leprosy books. It was hard to find any hope of cure in the texts. It was accepted that attempts at cure were completely useless. Amputation was usually recommended – but we knew that that produced still worse problems – as illustrated by Ah Tung in chapter 9.

From about that time I began regularly visiting the government outpatient clinics, on a Wednesday afternoon, to see patients and follow up those whom we had discharged, and also to do longer term follow-ups on these feet. I observed that the bones, if adequately protected, did heal and would remain healed for several years at least – so why not for life?

In 1960 I had realized that, in leprosy, some fractured foot bones **would** heal. Now I was realizing that we could significantly improve the shape and function of feet that had become deformed as a result of these fractures. Also I was learning the factors that might result in problems and fractures. To me it was all in the day's work in helping these patients.

There was one patient, Ah Lau, who had, one after the other, three fractures in the same foot, none due to severe trauma, and each a different bone. His case taught us more significant facts. We showed that once these fractured bones do heal, they are much tougher than normal bone and more difficult to fracture. I have never seen the same bone fracture twice. But while in the cast, the surrounding non-fractured bones weaken and so are more vulnerable to fracture.

We were collecting a lot of very interesting information about these bones in nerve damaged feet and we had the X-rays to show what was happening. In 1967 Dr James Isbister, one of my tutors when I was a medical student, visited the island, and I realized the importance of what we were observing. He spent a long time looking at the X-rays and checking the histories. He was fascinated. He was a physician and understood why the bones were weakening. His experience enabled him to correlate it to many other medical conditions. This was not a leprosy problem – it was general medicine.

Then he said, "You have enough material here to write a thesis for Doctor of Medicine (MD)". Though no academic, I knew that to be granted an MD one needed to produce a thesis proving something new, something not previously demonstrated. I had never expected to find something worth writing up for an MD degree. But then he added, "No, I do not think the Professor of Medicine would give an MD on a purely clinical thesis, but perhaps the Professor of Surgery will accept it for a Master of Surgery (MS), which is academically equivalent to an MD. I will approach him when I get back to Sydney." Eventually the letter came back from Australia: "Yes,

Professor John Lowenthal will allow you to submit it for Master of Surgery. You will need to apply direct to him."

I was then working with an elderly British radiologist, Dr Stephen Sturton, who reported on our chest X-rays. I told him about James' suggestion and the possibility of submitting a thesis. "Ah, yes," he said "You certainly have enough material to prove you can treat these bone problems adequately, but make sure you apply to present for the MS *in absentia.* If they will accept it *in absentia* they cannot call you in for oral examination." In an oral exam they could ask me about any aspect of surgery they liked – but, he said, "if they accept the thesis *in absentia* the whole degree stands or falls on that thesis." I could see the wisdom of that. As there were many areas of surgery that I knew nothing about, it would be very easy for me to be failed.

So I applied and in 1968 was accepted to do the MS *in absentia.* I was to get on with collecting my information and statistics and with writing the thesis, then when in Australia on leave I would discuss it with a supervisor to be appointed by the University. I went on leave in 1970. On arrival I met the professor who was to supervise me. He read what I had hopefully thought of as a final draft but told me that I had done it all the wrong way. I had to reorganize and rewrite it and virtually to start all over again – another year's work.

Several doctors who were visiting me for leprosy experience helped to check the manuscript – a massive job in the days before computers, when even photocopiers were a rarity. It meant carbon copies, typing and endless retyping. Our secretary had the job of typing two sets with carbons to make the required ten copies of the final thesis. Dozens of black and white photos also had to be printed and inserted, and all the copies bound. Eventually, in 1971 our copies were posted down to Sydney University.

Other than an acknowledgement of its arrival, I heard nothing about it for ages. Then one day, while visiting Singapore, I was racing across the compound at the General Hospital when I heard a familiar voice – "Oh, Dr Warren, I haven't seen you for a long time." It was Professor Pillay, Professor of Orthopaedics at the local Medical School, with whom I had worked on many occasions. I had taught him some of our techniques for tendon transfers in the hands. The surgeons I worked with at the Trafalgar Hospital had all been trainees under him. I replied "Well, yes sir, I have been very busy. I have been travelling a lot". He said "That was an excellent thesis". I flicked an eyebrow. I had no idea who had been asked to mark it. Sydney University had asked for four copies to be "marked by four people with appropriate experience".

He went on "I have asked that my copy be placed in the local Medical School library as an example of how a clinical thesis ought to be written. You do have your fellowship of the Royal Australasian College of Surgeons, do not you?" I replied "Well, no sir, I do not." His answer came "Well, you should have – I will see you again." And our ways parted as he had a clinic, and I had patients to see.

Finally in 1972 I was awarded the degree of Master of Surgery (University of Sydney). I gleaned on the grapevine that the university had no staff member who was experienced in the topic of my thesis, so they needed to rely on external examiners. Copies were sent to Dr Paul Brand, my original mentor, to Professor Pillay with whom I had worked in Singapore, and to Professor Donald Gunn who had worked at the Sungei Buloh leprosy hospital. So now I had come round through the back door and achieved a post graduate surgical degree! This was thanks to the mass of material I had accumulated as I helped leprosy patients. I thanked God too for the powers of observation, logic and resourcefulness he had given me.

There was more to come. I received a phone call on Hay Ling Chau early in 1973. It was from the professor of surgery at Hong Kong University. "Ah. Good morning, Dr Warren. I have a group of medical students that I would like to bring out for you to show what you are doing for leprosy. Could I bring them, say, next Tuesday?" I agreed to that. "Well", he said, "Would you by any chance be operating that afternoon? I would like to see some of your surgery. Could you put the students on the return boat at lunch time so we can operate in the afternoon?" It was all amusingly polite and indirect.

I organized to do one of the hand operations that Paul Brand had perfected and that I regarded as one of my show pieces. It was a beautiful procedure technically, as well as being post-operatively functional. We did so many that the staff knew the procedure well. For courtesy's sake, as we were getting organized and I had started the anaesthesia, I asked if he wished to scrub in and assist. "Well," he said, "That would be nice. I have been asked by the Australasian College to come and see your work."

That was a sudden surprise. I managed to let Kathleen Collett, who was also in the operating room, know what was happening so that she could pray for us! As it happened everything went beautifully – no problems – and I am sure he was quite impressed. I guess that this report was a vital factor in my being granted an Elected Fellowship of the Royal Australasian College of Surgeons. I did not actually receive it till 1977. These events started the ball rolling for me to receive further medical and academic recognition. Such news filters through the medical fraternity. When next in Australia (1974) I was asked to see patients with similar problems due to conditions other than leprosy, and to operate on some of them.

13

Surgical Dreams Realized

The first operation I was involved in on Hay Ling Chau was for an old lady with a broken hip. A professor of orthopaedics came over on a Saturday to pin her leg and I gave an anaesthetic. The operation was a success and the patient lived with us for many years.

From then on I did anaesthetics, while Dr Harman did the surgery. After a while I realised that a lot of the surgery did not require a general anaesthetic. Having learnt the basics of anaesthetics in Australia, I soon discovered that I could administer adequate anaesthesia under 'local blocks'. So I started doing some operations myself.

In our doctors' library there were plenty of reference books. There were always people to correspond with who would give suggestions and ideas. So I started doing some of the reconstructive surgery in 1959. I had always wanted to do surgery and so it was wonderful to be realising my dream, with plenty of patients waiting. They soon realised the potential and the requests that I received were diverse and fascinating, such as, "New eyelashes, please"; or "Please pin my ears back"! We strictly limited our attempts to the problems caused by leprosy, and I personally would only attempt new things if I thought that I would not make the patient any worse!

In Korea I had done quite a bit of surgery, often caesarean sections – sometimes life-saving emergencies with high drama. Now it was all elective surgery. I could select the timing to suit myself and the patient's general condition. There was time to plan, to think what I was going to do, and, more importantly, to think about the patient's long-term quality of life, because the point of doing rehabilitation surgery is to improve the patient's ability to care for him or herself. And so began my life-long dream – surgery.

Of course a surgeon needs a lot of extra knowledge. I have already mentioned that I had to learn physiotherapy. I also had to learn how to apply plaster casts, because, as a resident medical officer in Australia, I had had little chance to practise that skill. Dr Paul Brand had discovered that applying a plaster cast over an ulcer on a foot will usually produce healing within six to eight weeks. It was not necessary to change the dressing daily or the cast. The patient could walk and continue his everyday life without the need to be admitted to hospital.

I soon became expert at putting casts on with various foot pieces that enabled a patient to walk. Some were metal, called "Bohler irons", to lift the foot off the ground and take the patient's weight on the leg, not the foot. There were other methods too; I needed to become familiar with them all, and to find what suited our patients best.

Deformities of the hands and feet are those most amenable to correction by surgery. Deformed feet cause tragic hardships worldwide, but especially in undeveloped areas – in paddy fields or rough terrain and where people have to walk long distances.

Paul Brand had realised that there was a muscle (tibialis posterior) on the back of the leg which, in leprosy patients, was very rarely affected by the disease. It is possible to transfer the tendon of that muscle removing it from its original insertion on the inside of the heel, swinging it around the leg, and fixing it onto the top (the dorsum) of the foot. As a result when the patient thinks that he is turning his heel in – because that is the main function of the tibialis posterior muscle – he will be raising his foot at the ankle, producing the needed hinge movement. We then teach the patient by physiotherapy to integrate that action with his walking. I first started doing this type of surgery at Hay Ling Chau in 1959. I did a lot of tendon transfers, mostly with encouraging results. I was learning on the job. I also made various adaptations of the original method that were far more suitable for our patients and allowed them to start walking sooner. Our adaptation also reduced the chance of those disintegrating fractures such as Chung's (Chapter 9) that were occurring after some methods of foot-drop correction.

I also developed the art of tendon transfers to restore function in hands, and with the new intensive physiotherapy program the results were obviously better – although we had to wait a few years to be sure that the results would last. By the time I visited Paul Brand in India I was already regularly getting good results. Also Dr Goodwin had passed on surgical tips he had learnt. It was most rewarding to see both the restoration of ability and the response of the patients.

In 1963 while on leave in Australia, I was talking with a group of surgeons about reconstructing the anaesthetic hands of leprosy patients. One of them said, "You cannot do tendon transfers on an anaesthetic hand – it is a waste of time. They'll never learn to use it because they cannot feel." Well, by experience I knew better. There is just no logic in that statement, because you do not move by feel. A patient can *see* what he's meant to do and then learn to do it. It is more difficult if the patient is blind and has nerve damage in his hands.

The possibilities of reconstructive surgery became fascinating and exciting. It was still in its early days when I went to Hong Kong. No specialist was doing this type of work. Within a few years I was receiving requests to operate on non-leprosy patients in Hong Kong. Local surgeons were asking to come to the island to operate with me so they could learn. Above all I was always trying to find newer and better ways of improving the function of the hands and feet of the patients.

The next stage in my surgical dream developed rather unexpectedly. As I returned to Hong Kong in mid 1964, I stopped over in Singapore and Kuala Lumpur and visited the local leprosy hospitals. I was warmly welcomed in other places. In Singapore the superintendent showed me some of the patients' problems. He asked my opinion about one woman with a twisted foot. I recommended an operation to straighten it. The patient said, "When?". The superintendent was amazed. He said that several surgeons had previously suggested operating but the patient had always said "No". The superintendent then suggested that I return to Singapore when the new operation room was completed in 1965 to teach Government doctors and the other staff how to do the surgery. Visiting plastic surgeons had been working but the results were not consistently good.

From Singapore, I took a quick flight to Kuala Lumpur and visited my old school friend, Kathleen Collett, who lived in one of the resettlement villages. These were built in the 1950s when communist insurgents and rebels often attacked the small villages, seeking supplies. New, larger villages were set up, and people were moved into these settlements which were guarded against terrorists and bandits who might attack at night. Gates were shut from sundown till sunrise.

I stayed with Kathleen, who was doing general nursing in a new village just north of Kuala Lumpur near the big Government leprosy hospital, Sungei Buloh. As I was interested in leprosy work, Kathleen arranged for a church friend who worked at the hospital, John Pearson, to collect me and take me there. He was doing drug trials for leprosy for the UK Medical Research Council.

At the leprosarium we joined a routine weekly ward round. Within an hour or so, however, a couple of the doctors interested in surgery came and asked me if I could go and see some surgical patients. The upshot was that they asked me to operate that afternoon on two of their patients. So on my very first day in Sungei Buloh, I spent the afternoon in the operating theatre!

The doctors were so thrilled to have someone to come and help that the superintendent, Dr Bjowani, a lovely Indian surgeon, begged me to come back in the future. They presented me with a huge bunch of purple orchids grown by the patients. I flew back into Hong Kong the next day with them. The odd thing was that, when I left Kuala Lumpur, those orchids were purple, and still purple when I got back to Hong Kong that night. But by the next morning they were white! Why? I have never found an answer, nor seen that colour change again, and I have carried orchids in planes many times since.

I now had requests to go to Singapore and Sungei Buloh, to teach surgery. First however I needed to ensure the Chinese doctors were able to run Hay Ling Chau, and I had to convince TLM that this was the way of the future and that Hay Ling Chau could do without me for a few weeks at a time. This was the sort of thing I had dreamed of when I visited Taiwan in 1960. God could open doors if it was his will. By 1965 Dr Goodwin had returned to England, but the two Chinese doctors and staff could carry on the work while I was away – so long as it was not for too long!

The mission wanted me to attend the Pan-Pacific Conference on the Rehabilitation of the Disabled, to be held in Tokyo in April of 65, at which there would be a special section for leprosy. Our physiotherapist, Jean Watson, was also invited, and was asked to run a workshop before the conference for physiotherapists in the Japanese leprosy hospitals. They were mostly masseurs; we wanted to teach them to get patients working themselves as we had found the patients could do so much by self-care to help themselves. Jean lectured and taught along those lines while I spent a couple of days at the leprosy hospital teaching reconstructive surgery. At the conference's special leprosy session I read a paper, and we had also prepared a series of posters on patient self-care and how they could protect themselves from injury. This I think was one of the main messages that those of us working at Hay Ling Chau were trying to get across in those days – saving hands and feet for future usefulness. We taught self help – how much they could do for themselves – and how, and why. This gave the patients a sense of purpose and optimism about their future.

The Japanese Leprosy Association treated Jean and me to a weekend at Lake Hakone almost at the foot of Mt Fujiyama. They footed all the bills – a lovely unexpected extra. We shared a room overlooking the lake. I woke just at dawn and could not resist waking Jean to see the glorious sunrise lighting the peak of Mt Fuji. She grumbled, but later thanked me for pushing her to take a photo which came out beautifully. We also attended a conference dinner, at which I sat opposite the brother of the Emperor of Japan. When I wrote this to my mother she replied that, due to my swelled head, she would now have to throw out all my hats! This trip indeed showed that the Chinese doctors were able to maintain the general and medical program on Hay Ling Chau while I was away. So I received the go-ahead to travel regularly to the leprosy hospitals in Malaya and Singapore.

Jean Watson and I commenced this routine in September 1965. I would fly out from Hong Kong to Kuala Lumpur. There I would see patients, advise, and select for surgery. The next day I would operate with colleagues, and continue surgery for 7-10 days. I would then depart for Singapore, leaving instructions about the post-operative physiotherapy requirements. Jean Watson would travel there three or four weeks later, remove the plaster casts and start the follow-up therapy, teaching the local physiotherapists how to continue it. In Singapore I would work for another seven or ten days of surgery and teaching. Jean would come on from Kuala Lumpur and make sure that the patients there were getting the right post-operative care.

Then came a hectic trip into Thailand, for which I could only obtain a 48-hour visa. I would catch an early morning flight to

Bangkok where a car waited to rush me to Manorom for a ward round. The next day would be spent in the operating room, and, leaving full instructions for follow-up, I would depart at 3 am to get to Bangkok to catch the early plane to Hong Kong!

We were able to maintain this program over the next few years, going to Malaysia, Singapore and Thailand every three or four months. At times exhausting, it was nevertheless rewarding. We met lots of patients who had been operated on by other surgeons – surgeons from various countries of the world – quite often fully accredited "proper" plastic surgeons. Very few of them understood about the problems of the completely anaesthetic limb. Often, with no physiotherapy re-education instruction, the patient never learnt to use the transfer.

In 1965 I visited South Korea for the first time since 1959, to visit the relatively new TLM hospital built in the university campus at Taegu. This hospital had developed out of the mobile clinic program that I had originally seen in 1958. The hospital was set up and managed by non-medical TLM personnel with the medical component supplied by the university medical staff and locally employed doctors. The mission was keen that I go back there to help them with the medical work. It was now a well established program and I had the chance of teaching techniques. That was the first of many trips to help in the Korean program.

So doors opened up. It was deeply satisfying to be part of the program of making Paul Brand's work known in the places where it was most needed, and taking it further. Others were coming to Hay Ling Chau to learn. In 1967 I was asked to go and teach in Pakistan. [See chapter 10.] Again, there were hundreds of patients almost untouched by the hope and possibility of reconstructed limbs, and I was given the opportunity to lead the way. I have a poster on my wall. "*Do not follow where the path may lead. Go instead where there is no path and leave a trail.*" I had no idea at that stage of how far the trail would go, or how many lives would be touched by the ways God was leading me to develop and apply the abilities he'd given me.

In February 1967, after six weeks' leave in Australia, I visited Kuching (East Malaysia) Leprosy Hospital on the way to Hong Kong. Dr Fraser's experiment in setting up Hay Ling Chau was certainly paying off. Not only were we discharging many patients who had benefited from rehabilitation and reconstructive surgery, but our work was touching many others in the Asian area.

This was the time when I was assessing our Hong Kong results, and especially the work on bone problems and starting on the research for my thesis. It was a period of real achievement and consolidation, culminating in my being invited to organize and chair the section on Leprosy at the Pan Pacific Conference for Rehabilitation of the Disabled, held in Hong Kong in 1968, just before I went to London.

In the following years, 1969-70, both the travelling and the thesis work continued. The numbers of patients on the island were falling and we were admitting fewer for surgery. Now that the leprosy situation was under control the government was keen to close the institution and admit any patients who needed care to their hospital in Kowloon. So our work load slowly decreased until the Government decided on closure at the end of 1974.

14

DRUG TRIAL – LAMPRENE IN ACTION

In 1968, sponsored by Ciba-Geigy, the manufacturers of the leprosy drug Lamprene, I was able to attend an International Leprosy Congress in London. This was my first visit to England. I was to deliver a paper as part of their multi-centric trial of the drug. The Ciba medical group (now Novartis) were supplying us with the drug which we first knew as CIBA1906 and then as B663; it later became known as clofazimine and now finally by its trade name, Lamprene. Derived from safranine, the bright yellow food dye used for colouring saffron rice, amongst other things, this drug was developed in Ireland in the early 1950s, when it was discovered that in mice it was effective against tuberculosis. When it was tried against human tuberculosis (TB) it did not work as hoped, because the TB bacillus in humans does not actually live inside the cells as it does in mice. But the leprosy germ is an intracellular organism: it lives and multiplies inside the macrophage cells that ingest it to destroy it. Lamprene has the ability to get into those cells and stay there and destroy any organisms that are eaten by the macrophage cells. It can actually eliminate the infection of leprosy in humans.

The leprosy expert Dr Stanley Browne, working in Africa, was one of the first to use Lamprene on any scale. He found that the drug increases the rate the leprosy organisn is killed with fewer undesirable side-effects than other medications. He was convinced that this was an effective drug that needed to be used more. Its use allowed him to make a long step forward in the treatment of leprosy. The drug company Ciba therefore organised a large multi-centre trial in which a number of people like me, who were dealing with many sufferers from lepromatous leprosy, were given large quantities of Lamprene and told to use it for lepromatous and near-lepromatous – that is, low resistance – leprosy patients, people whose bodies lack the ability to eliminate the bacteria.

Drug trials need to test any new drug on hard cases. People who develop the lepromatous form of leprosy have a very low ability to eliminate the bacteria spontaneously. The bacteria may live in their bodies for many, many years and slowly multiply. It may be up to twenty or more years before any obvious clinical sign of the disease appears. However, it will slowly progress until there are literally millions of the leprosy bacteria. If a drug could be shown to be effective with these low resistance cases, it would demonstrate a genuine breakthrough. In another form of the disease known as tuberculoid leprosy, there is a natural potential for patients to get rid of the bacteria themselves. For trials it was important to select the most severe non-self-healing patients, so that no-one could say that the good results could have happened anyway, without treatment.

Another complicating factor is that when the leprosy bacteria are killed, an antigen is liberated from the capsule of the organism. In leprosy the antigen itself does not do any real harm, but when it is present the body's immune system recognises it as a foreign protein that must be eliminated producing antibodies which will combine with the antigen to neutralise it. This is a mechanism which our bodies use in many circumstances to get rid of unwanted proteins, such as antigens from pollen – as in people who have asthma; or from food that we eat – as in children with peanut allergies. Antigens that are adequately neutralised by antibodies will usually not produce medical problems.

Unfortunately, in leprosy, when the leprosy antigen is neutralised by the patient's antibody, the molecule that is formed is rather a large one, so large in fact that it gets stuck in small blood vessels and produces an inflammatory response in them – a "vasculitis". Once the bacteria are being killed adequately in lepromatous leprosy patients, they may start getting little red spots on the skin which we call erythema nodosum leprosum: ENL for short. A few ENL are no problem to anybody. If there are a lot of ENL, the patient may feel generally sick and miserable, and may develop high fevers and is said to have lepra reaction. Those little pink spots are usually of nuisance value only, but may in fact ulcerate and become infected. So we need special treatment to look after these people. Many of the severe complications of leprosy are due to the effect of ENL in the nerves and eyes and in other parts of the body where the antigen has collected, because previously there have been many leprosy bacilli in that site.

Once Lamprene gets into the cells it is effective in killing the leprosy bacilli. The number of bacilli will stop increasing and the population of bacteria in that patient's body will slowly fall. Lamprene also affects ENL, dramatically reducing the severity of the lepra reaction, and having an anti-inflammatory effect.

In the mid-sixties Dr Stanley Browne, TLM medical adviser at that time, visited our work in Hong Kong and saw some patients with chronic ENL. Some of them had been given corticosteroids years earlier and were now virtually dependent on steroids. I could not get them off the drug; every time I tried to reduce the dose they would complain of new symptoms and other complications. It is possible to buy steroids over the counter in many less developed countries. The steroids often make people "feel good". If we have given the patient a taste of the euphoria that often accompanies the use of steroids we may in fact have contributed to making that patient drug-dependent – addicted to steroids. So particularly in third world countries where the giving and taking of drugs cannot be adequately supervised, I do not like giving steroids. I am well aware that lots of people do give them, and there are situations in which I do also, but in this particular type of leprosy I prefer to keep patients off steroids if possible. I really felt in a cleft stick. Stanley appreciated this and said after he saw my patients, "I will see if Ciba-Geigy will give you some of this drug Lamprene for a drug trial. It will help get them off their steroids."

Soon after that our first batch arrived. The first patient I gave it to was a young woman, a very intelligent girl who was a school teacher, but at that stage had no real deformity. She did have bad ENL. She was meant to be teaching the children at Hay Ling Chau but unfortunately she had to spend time in hospital because lepra reaction made her so sick. When the Lamprene came and we put her on it, within a couple of months she was fine – no more ENL problems! She was back at school, full time, teaching the children. As long as she could remain on the drug she remained well until her disease was controlled. We reported the good results to Ciba-Geigy, so they then included us in their big drug trial. We ended up with literally dozens of these patients with chronic ENL and other forms of reaction, receiving Lamprene free of charge from Ciba-Geigy. We had to experiment to find out the best dosage for each patient. Some only needed 50 milligrams daily; some up to 300 milligrams. But it certainly did make a very big difference to the patients who had had an unpleasant ENL reaction for a long time.

What Stanley Browne discovered and what I was then able to confirm, was that when we put a patient on Lamprene the number of ENL dropped quite dramatically. Quoting the results we had with the drug trials we were doing, I wrote and presented a paper at the London conference in 1968, and later had it published.

Once we got some of my patients in Hong Kong who were chronic sufferers from ENL onto an adequate dose of Lamprene, they stopped getting ENL completely, and the number of bacilli in their bodies fell more rapidly than previously. So Lamprene turned out to be a drug which not only treated the infection but helped to control and treat a lot of its complications.

There was one major drawback. The dye in the drug is deposited into the leprosy lesions and turns the skin quite dark in many patients. With the diffuse type of skin lesions the skin colour would be fairly uniform, like a good suntan, but if they had obvious skin patches with clear-cut edges these patches could become very dark. Hence Lamprene can make the disease more obvious. The Chinese admire light-coloured skin; they do not like to get suntanned and they do not like the pigmentation produced by Lamprene. But if they really do understand their problems and the effectiveness of Lamprene they will agree to take the drug. We can reassure them that the colour will slowly fade once the drug is discontinued.

From my observation, the use of Lamprene had resulted in a marked drop in the incidence of difficult reaction cases. It is now given routinely as part of the Multi-Drug Therapy (MDT) that the World Health Organisation recommends, and it seems that its regular inclusion has even reduced the total number of those developing reaction. If I only had one drug for leprosy I would choose Lamprene.

So essentially what I have related above is the report I gave at the conference in London, which was a real success. I met many of the top names in leprosy and made many new friends. As usual there were opportunities to discuss mutual problems and to find out how other people tackled them.

Ciba generously kept us well supplied with Lamprene so that I could go on treating as many as I deemed suitable until Hay Ling Chau closed in 1975. As a result, we were able to supply Ciba with the records of many patients supporting the use of Lamprene for treating "lepra reaction of the ENL type". Over the next decade Lamprene became much more popular, and WHO included it as one of the main drugs in the treatment of leprosy when it published its MDT recommendations. One very interesting fact is that, although the leprosy bacillus has a marked ability to become resistant to almost every drug we try to roll at it to knock it out, now, some 30 years later, we have still not seen the organism in a leprosy patient develop resistance to Lamprene given routinely (although a resistant strain was eventually produced in a laboratory.)

The Congress in London was a key time in the use of Lamprene. Ciba-Geigy sponsored a large number of those conducting their trials, like myself, to attend and special sessions were held about this new drug. Since it has far fewer side effects than many other drugs, many of us are convinced that it is currently the safest anti-leprosy drug available.

So as clinical researchers back in 1968, we had a good opportunity to compare our protocols and design variations in medication. Of course many other topics were discussed; I was especially interested in the progress in reconstructive surgery and the use of plaster casts for ulcer care. By this time Paul Brand's pioneering work in this method of treatment had become widely adopted in the leprosy endemic world and so we were comparing results in different situations.

15

Chiang Mai – The King and I

I had visited Chiang Mai in NW Thailand briefly in 1962 after I had been working in Manorom Hospital for several weeks. I saw a few tourist sights and then was shown around the McKean Institute. (See chapter 10) About a thousand patients lived on an island in the River Ping, that in 1907 had been given to the Presbyterian Church by the Thai king. The patients lived in simple but adequate thatched houses and looked after themselves as far as possible.

At that time little or no rehabilitation surgery was done and there was no regular physiotherapy or teaching of prevention of deformity. There was an ulcer clinic but I think that was about all. In the next decade Dr John Bissett, a Canadian surgeon, was appointed. He did some training in India and started reconstructive surgery and the necessary ancillary programs.

In 1969 Dr Trevor Smith and his wife Heather from Australia were appointed and came to Hay Ling Chau en route to McKean to learn the basics of leprosy from us. Trevor's brief was to learn the medical aspects of leprosy, not surgery, as John Bissett was the surgeon. Trevor would be required to give anaesthetics to enable John to operate.

Some months after they arrived in Chiang Mai I visited and learnt a little more of how McKean functioned and what John was doing. I did a few procedures with John. Subsequently I had little to do with McKean until after I moved to Manorom. Then John announced that he was leaving, migrating to New Zealand so that his son could train there as a doctor.

Trevor was to take over as Chief Medical Officer. The Thai superintendent was not a medical person, so I was asked if I could

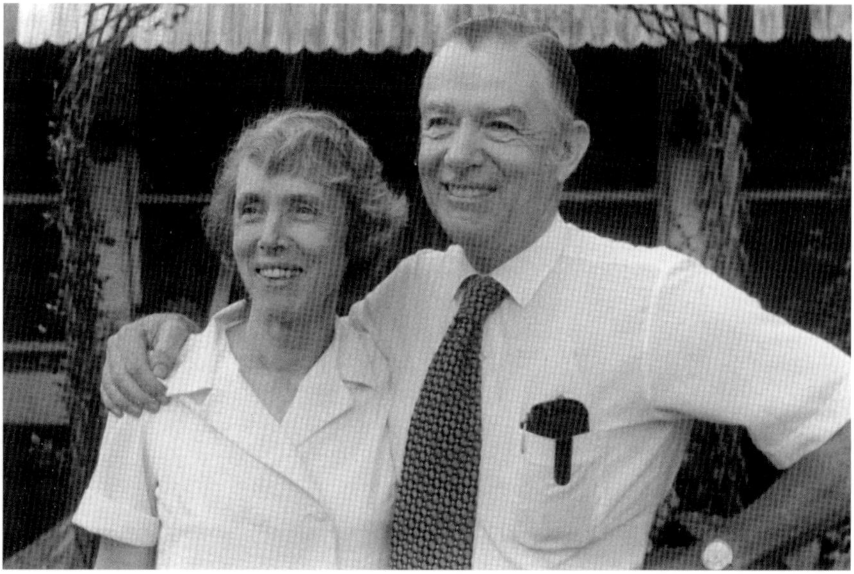

Dr Paul Brand and Dr Margaret Brand

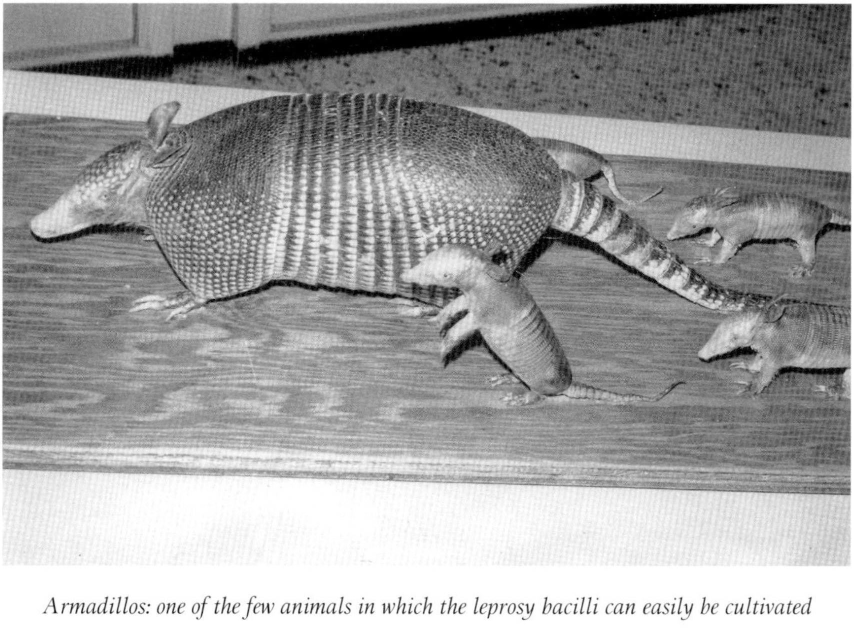

Armadillos: one of the few animals in which the leprosy bacilli can easily be cultivated

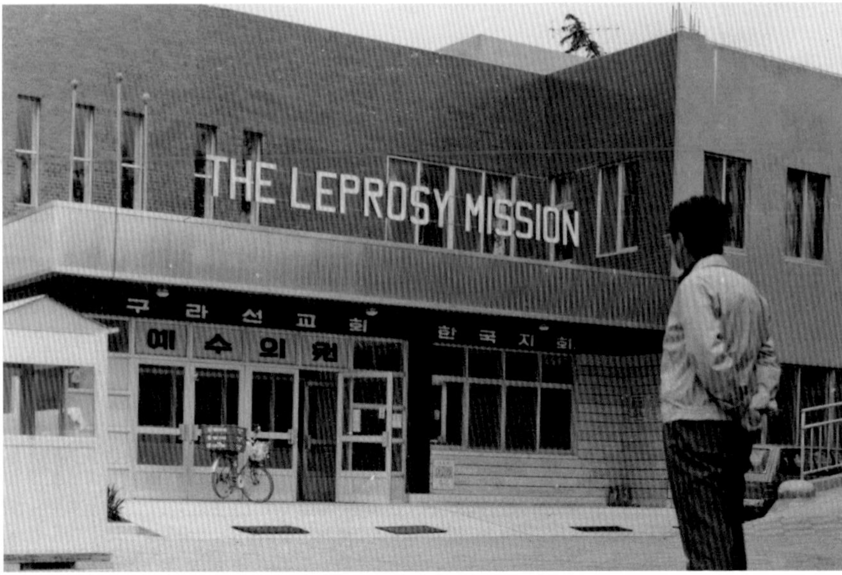

The Leprosy Mission Hospital - Taegu, South Korea

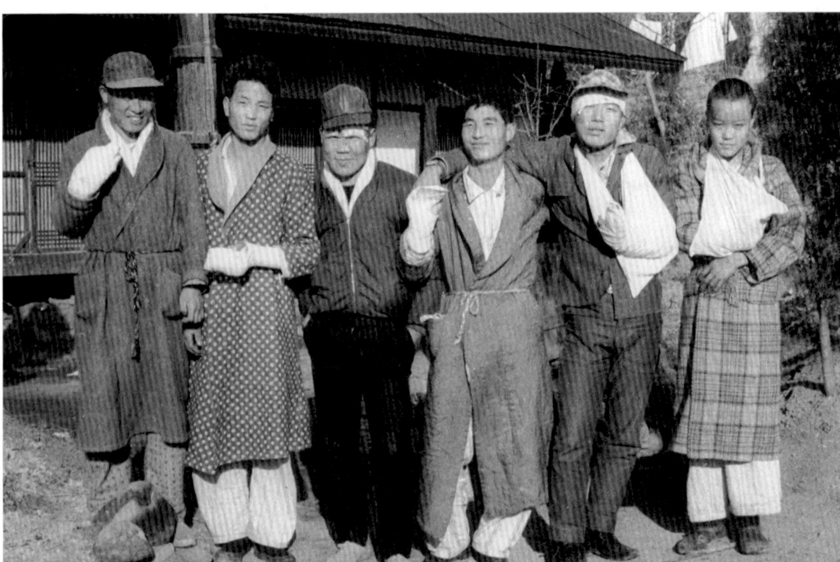

Korean patients after surgery. Note eyebrow dressings and plaster casts on hands

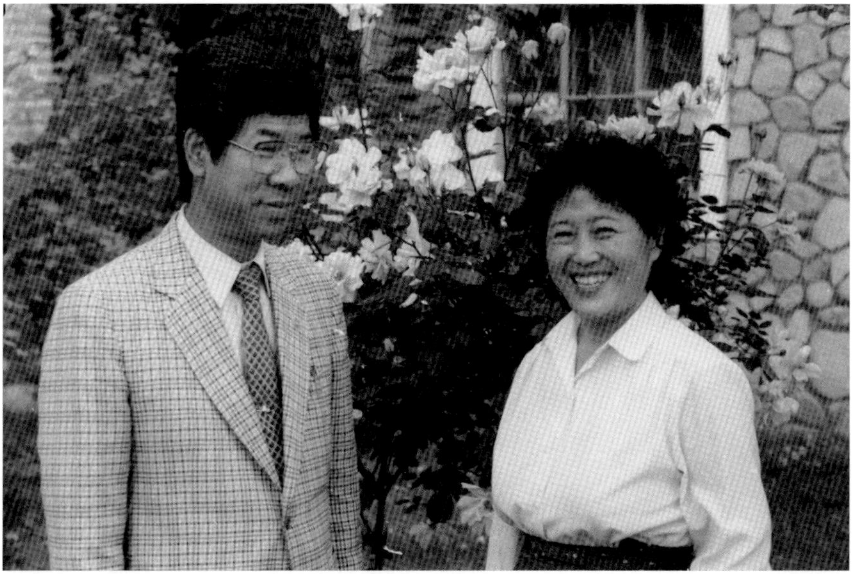

Mr Cho (administrator) and his wife (head nurse) at TLM – Taegu, South Korea 1983

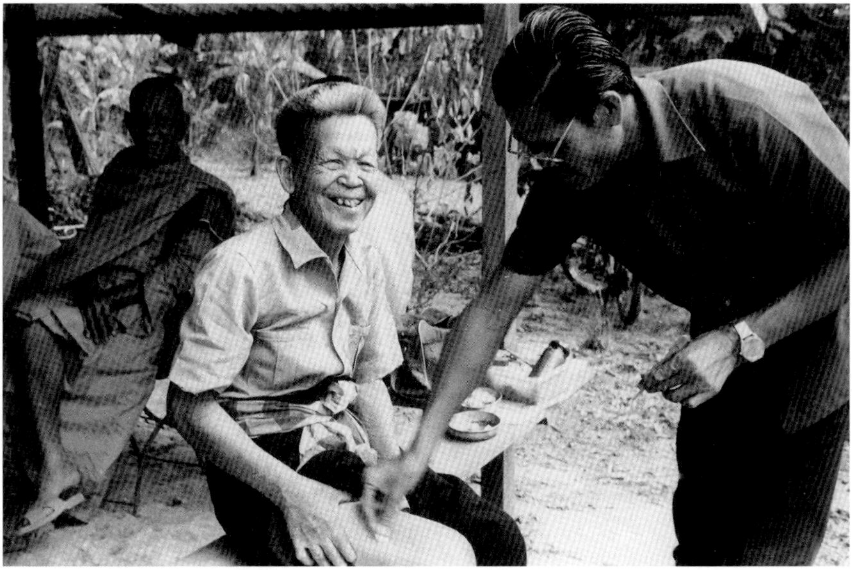

Skin smear being taken from leprosy patient by paramedical worker at a 'Sala' clinic - Thailand

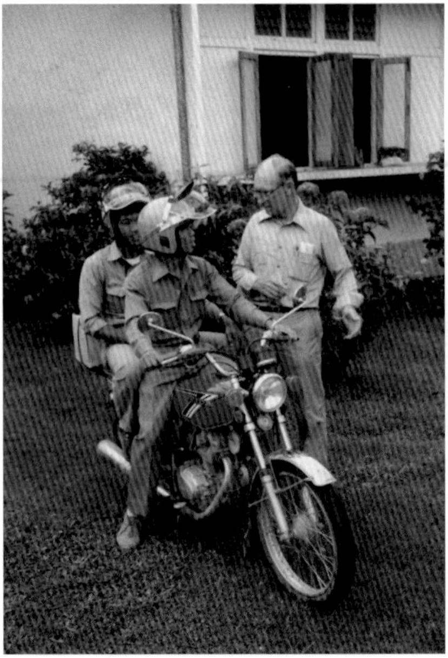

Alan Davis of TLM with two paramedical workers setting off on home visits - Manorom, Thailand

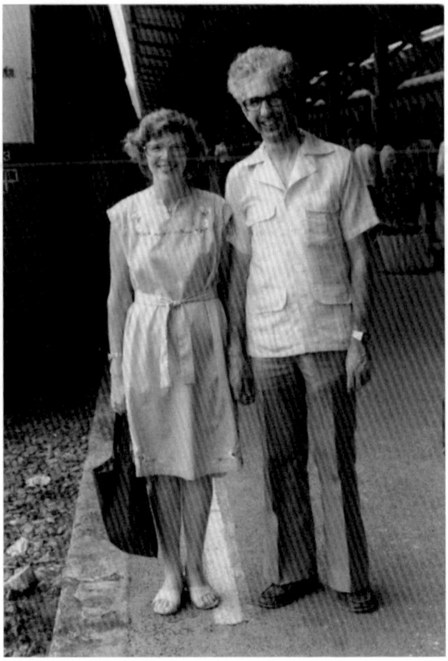

Dr Trevor & Mrs Heather Smith - Australians serving in Chiang Mai, Thailand

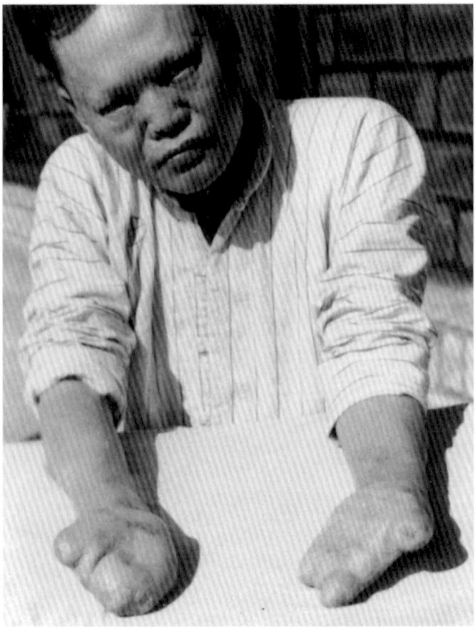

Mr Lum arrived with no fingers and no eyebrows: life is hard

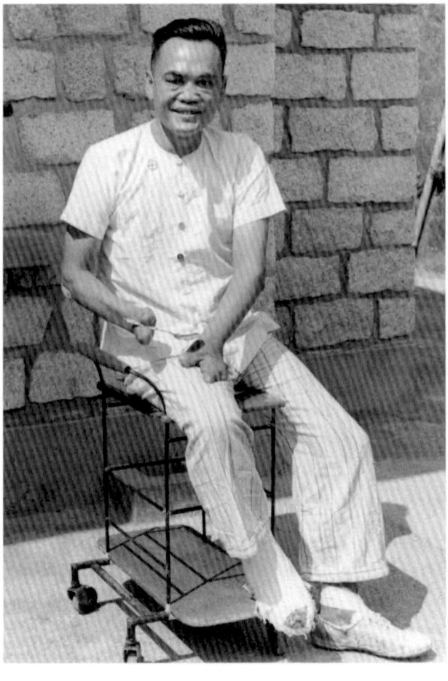

"Look; I can hold a spoon in one hand". New eyebrows, a hand which grips, and feet being treated.

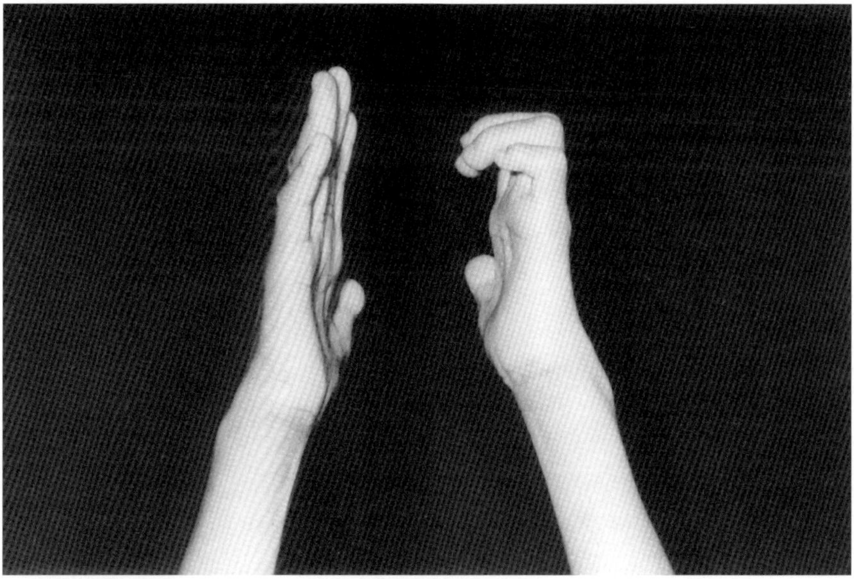

Jay Jay's hands after surgery to one hand, shows difference in finger position and straightness

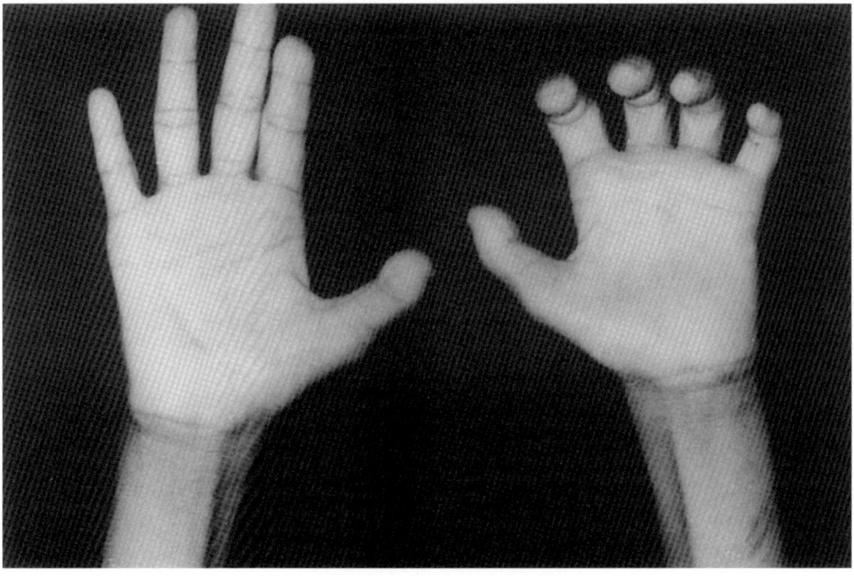

Palm view shows straightness of fingers and wider thumb web to give grasp

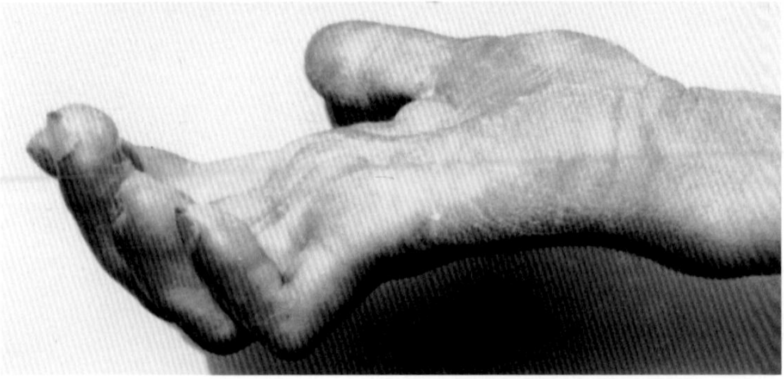

Typical clawed hand: fingers will not straighten, and thumb cannot lift out to pinch

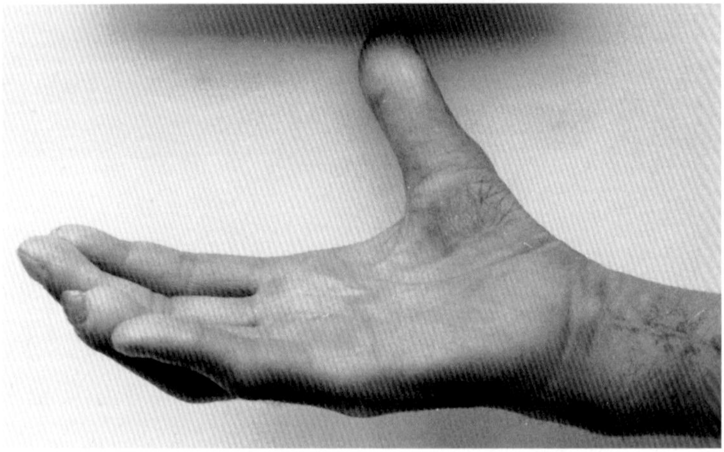

After surgery: straight fingers and a thumb which can pinch and grip

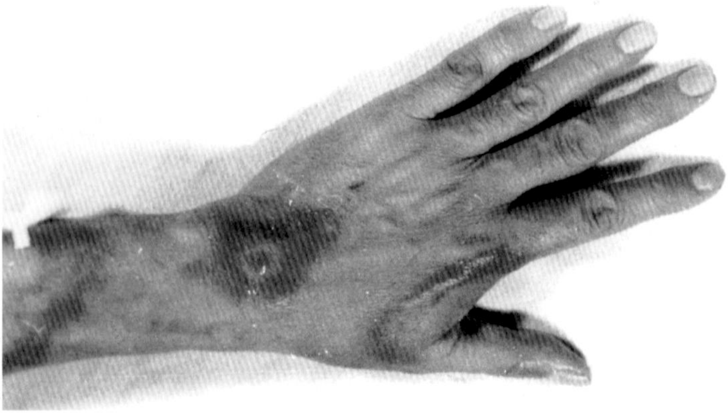

Typical borderline type of leprosy skin lesion

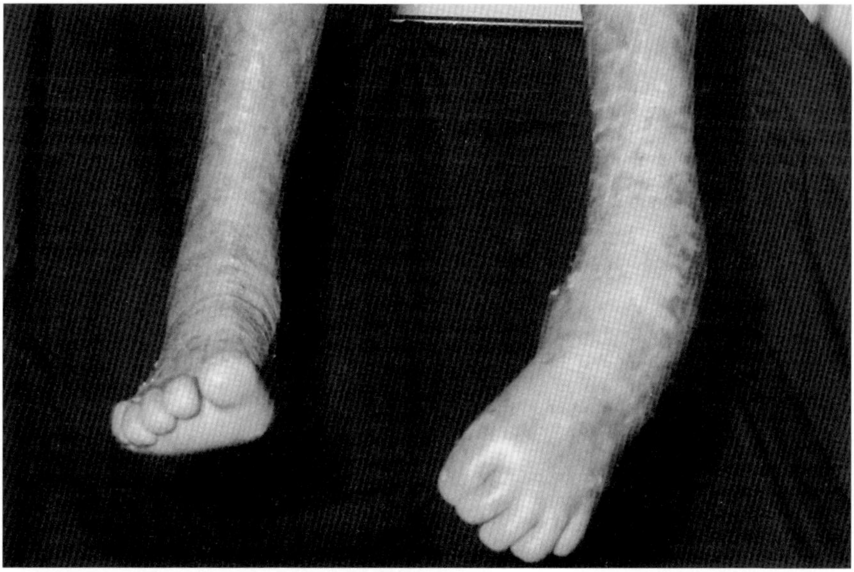

Left foot typically deformed and twisted - cannot walk

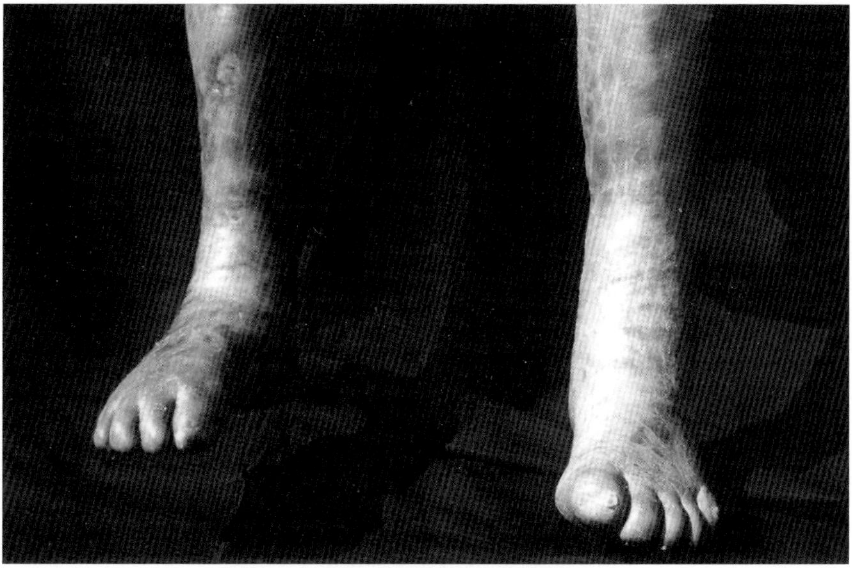

After surgery - can now walk and wear a shoe

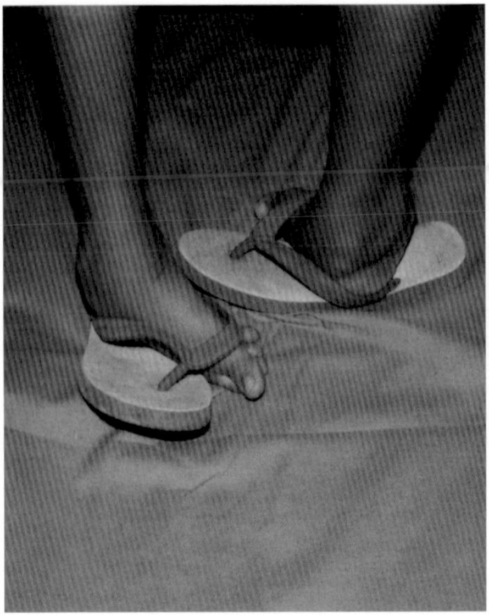

Congenital bilateral club feet in adult lady - no shoes will fit

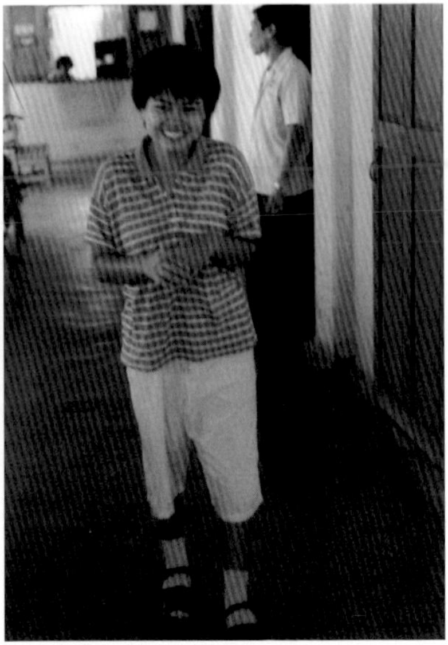

After surgery, patient thrilled to wear normal shoes, and walk

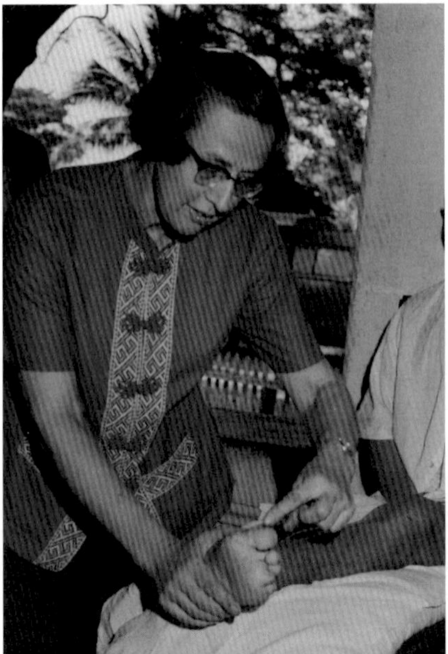

Dr Grace examining a foot

visit McKean regularly in order to continue the rehabilitation surgery that John had started. We agreed that that would be possible and practical since I now lived in Thailand. We also planned that Trevor Smith would to learn some of the surgery so that the common problems did not need to wait till I arrived. So from 1975 to 1989, while I was living at Manorom, I was going north to Chiang Mai regularly – sometimes every three or four months to do a week or ten days of work. I was able to teach Trevor to do quite a bit of surgery, and before long he could do the routine foot-drop corrections. He learnt how to clean up infected areas, especially abscesses, and to do amputations when necessary – though our rule was to save enough foot to walk on if at all possible.

When I first went to McKean, Trevor either gave the anaesthetic – if a general anaesthetic was required – or more typically, he assisted me with the type of local anaesthesia I generally used. Hence Trevor was able to do a lot of the surgery, but he left to me the more complicated problems – especially the hands and face reconstruction work.

In the 1970s, a number of plastic surgeons from other hospitals came and worked with us at McKean and the medical school because they soon realised that we provided a valuable source of teaching and learning material. So whenever I went, people came in to learn so they could do the same procedures themselves. It has been fascinating to reflect on the different students who have come to work with me. Some of them have been excellent, but some hardly knew which end of a knife to hold, and, sadly, would never be any good. I believe some people are born surgeons, some people you can make into surgeons, but some people will never be surgeons.

Many of them would also ask if I could help them get a scholarship to go and study surgery, or even just leprosy, overseas. Part of the reason, unfortunately, was not a desire to help the patient at all, but a desire for the kudos that they would receive if they were able to say that they had studied abroad. Living in a country like Australia, it is very difficult to appreciate the backgrounds from which many of our associates in the Third World come. Some of them desperately desire to gain status and prestige, to make a good impression on their fellow doctors and patients, and overseas study is one much sought-after way to achieve that.

In my earlier stays in India I saw notices saying that a person was a BA (failed)! Even that they had studied towards a BA was a big plus for some. That they had not passed the exams did not matter. This was also a problem with some of the people trained by TLM in simple leprosy therapy techniques. They have then put up their plates saying that they are fully qualified physiotherapists. Sadly, that is incorrect, and these people may earn the mission a bad name.

In the 1970s I encountered a teenager with badly deformed hands. It was a tragedy. While working he had been wading through water carrying a metal water pipe, when one end of the pipe touched a high tension cable. The burns left him with virtually no muscles or tendons on the front of both arms, from the wrist up towards the elbows. He had been taken to a major hospital in Chiang Mai where skin graft repairs had been done but had left him with absolutely rigid fingers, because he had no tendons to bend the joints to give him a grip. So one of the plastic surgeons brought him over to us to see what we could do for him.

Many operations followed over the next few years as we tried to help him. Most attempts to get the muscles to work again failed. Eventually we found a compromise. His fingers were stiff, but we were able to sneak a muscle in from the back of his arm to bend his fingers at the knuckles. This meant that he could, by bending his knuckles, bring his fingers down so that the tips touched the palm of his hand. In that way, we gave him some form of a grip. Sadly, there was no way we could get the thumb out and functioning normally, to give him a 'pinch' action. However, we did manage to move one of his muscles from the back of his arm and bring it around the side of his hand so it would hold the soft part of the thumb firmly against the side of the index finger. In doing this, we gave him what we call a "key grip". Key grips are very common in leprosy patients and we usually try to correct them, but in this young man it was the best we could achieve.

After about four or five years of work on his arms and hands, he left our surgical department and took his place with the many craftspeople who made and decorated lacquer objects. He was a lovely young man who eventually married another patient who also had real problems with her hands, but who had won through so that she could use them well.

In 1977 came the 70th anniversary of the founding of the McKean Institute in 1907 when the King of Thailand had given the island to the Presbyterians. We were informed that the present king (then and still in 2006) His Majesty King Bhumipol Adulyades was coming to celebrate with us. Oh, there was a great flurry! The Government even laid down some better roads for the event. That was a blessing – a good road surface was built not only in the grounds of the Institute but also to link the leprosarium to the main road.

A lot of protocol had to be observed. In Thailand, one always must respect the head: that is culturally important. If I need to examine a patient's face, I must sit down to look at him. If I need to touch his face, then I also need to apologise – a standard Thai apology which every foreigner must learn. When walking past someone seated one stoops to try to get lower than their head. In the capital Bangkok, people are relaxed about these things these days, but when you get out into the country areas, the need to respect a person's head still applies.

When it comes to the King, it is even more important. If you have seen the film *The King and I*, you might remember some lovely scenes in it, of people and staff literally on the floor as they bring their heads down lower than the King's. Basically, a Thai person never touches their monarch or his wife, the Queen. They do not shake hands with them; instead, they always bow with their hands together in a greeting called a *wai*, the standard Thai greeting.

When the King came to visit McKean, all the members of the staff had to be lined up. When he visited a building, the staff would be on the path outside as a 'Guard of Honour'. As he passed along, you would see each of them with their hands up doing the traditional *wai* and also bowing (or curtsying in the case of the women) trying to get their heads lower than his head.

So it was a very special day. Dr Trevor Smith and the Rev Dick Bryant (who was administrator at the time) were introduced to him. They did their *wais* and then he shook hands with them, because they were foreigners. Council members lined one path and one was an American well over six foot tall (in fact he was 200 cm!) There was no way he could get his head down low enough before the King. The King obviously did not mind – after all, he had studied abroad.

I was in the surgery block at that time and a whole group of elderly patients were brought in especially to see the King. They were sitting on mats on the floor lining the proposed path. They had no problem; their heads were well down below the King's, but it was interesting to see the way in which he and the Queen squatted while talking to the elderly patients who were sitting on the ground.

When the King met us, again he shook hands with the foreigners, but the Thais only greeted him with their traditional *wai* greeting and a bow. One of the Thai staff who was with us disintegrated into tears afterwards and said, "You touched our King! He shook hands with you, but we are never allowed to touch our monarch." It was moving to be put in a completely different category. Both the King and Queen chatted to us. She talked to me about the disabled and what we could do to help them. I do not know what the King talked to Trevor about – I guess there were a multitude of things, as Trevor escorted him for about an hour. He went around and saw the patients at work, and, at one stage, when he was in the lacquer-ware shop, he actually laid his hand on the shoulder of one of the patients. That was an overwhelming honour for the patient, and a very big thing for the King of Thailand to do. Another of the patients, an elderly disabled man who was working in one of the workshops, received a wonderful surprise. The King gave him a 500 baht note. (500 bahts then would have been worth about $ US10 or $12). This was not only an honour but unimaginable wealth!

The King and the Queen are really loved by their subjects. When I went back to Manorom Hospital and showed a photo of myself with the King and Queen, well, I'd really made it! That was something that every Thai person would have liked to have experienced – to be in a photo with the royal couple of Thailand!

McKean has changed a great deal over the years. Initially it was built just for leprosy patients when many of them needed somewhere to live. It has now become a Rehabilitation Centre for people suffering from lots of other disabilities and deformities. It is a place where they can receive proper physiotherapy and surgery. We have had the joy of seeing many patients restored to their families, enabled to look after themselves because of the corrective care and therapy we have been able to give at McKean. And so today after so many years, as it approaches its centenary, McKean is still evolving, and thankfully, the number of leprosy patients who need its special care is getting less and less. However, more and more non-leprosy patients are being referred for the intensive help that can be given. The patients come and go regularly – in for their surgery and rehabilitation and then home again.

On the island of McKean, besides the Leprosy Hospital, there is also what is called "The Northern Village". This was one of the villages where the patients used to live in the old days, but as the numbers of patients fell, it was decided that it should play a new role in the program. So the village was revamped, and now comprises little two-roomed houses where a couple of disabled people could live together, share the cooking and eating facilities and grow things in the small garden. Some of the houses were remodelled to remove the steps, allowing easier access for patients who were on crutches or in wheel chairs. The centre of the village became a type of community care centre with bed facilities where the disabled could be properly cared for, with physiotherapy provision. The village already had its own chapel. The King on his visit to McKean that day gave a substantial sum of money towards this village for the permanently disabled.

16

Round the World – 1

The year 1973 was the centenary of Armauer Hansen's discovery in Norway of the bacillus *Mycobacterium leprae* as the organism which causes leprosy.

This was quite a medical breakthrough because, until that time, it had not generally been realised that specific bacteria – of which there are hundreds of thousands of varieties – were the cause of many of the diseases that afflict humankind. It was Hansen that realised that the majority of leprosy patients that he was treating had these bacilli in their skin – so they were called Hansen's bacilli and were eventually recognised as the cause of the disease leprosy. Leprosy is often called Hansen's disease.

Some years later a scientist, Koch, realised that there were other bacteria that he was able to grow in cultures. It is now accepted that, to claim an organism causes a disease, it must be possible first to culture it, and then, by giving a dose, to give the same disease to another subject. Leprosy is one of the few diseases in which this has never been done in humans. We have been able to produce leprosy in laboratory animals – white mice and armadillos. But this is not the same as giving leprosy to a human being.

The reason for the difficulty in transmitting the disease to other people is partly that most humans have a natural resistance to leprosy. When a person is infected with leprosy bacilli, organisms may multiply in their body for a few weeks or months. Technically the person has caught it, but usually they are able to produce the right sort of cells – T-lymphocytes – which are capable of destroying the disease before there is any definite clinical sign of leprosy. One can say that these people have a sub-clinical disease; this is because we can find evidence in their bloodstream of these special T-lymphocytes produced by the body in order to kill the leprosy organisms circulating in the bloodstream.

Most people can develop these T-lymphocytes very rapidly. In the 1970s, there was a research project at the Leprosy Training Centre at Addis Ababa in Ethiopia. All the expatriates who came to work at that leprosy centre, who previously had never been in touch with leprosy, were checked on arrival for special T-lymphocytes. Before the end of that year, 80% of them, negative on arrival, had already caught leprosy – and had then cured themselves – as evidenced by the fact that T-lymphocytes were now in their blood. Once a person has an adequate number of T-lymphocytes, symptoms of leprosy are unlikely to develop.

So although a lot of people develop sub-clinical leprosy, very few (less than 5% of all people) develop clinical leprosy. Thus the finding by Hansen in 1873 that the majority of his 'active' patients had these organisms in their skin and in their nasal mucosa was not surprising.

1973 was the centenary of his work. So the International Leprosy Association changed the scheduled date of their big Congress from 1972 to 1973. The event was to be in Bergen, Norway, which was where Hansen had worked; the hospital was still there. It was now a museum, and we were able to visit it.

Since I had been doing research into the use of the new drug Lamprene, it was decided that I should go to this conference. I was due for furlough, so I would go to Bergen and then proceed home on leave, making various visits en route in order to see what was happening in other countries. I could teach and also speak at some TLM meetings.

This was going to be a long trip. Kathleen Collett had been working with me at Hay Ling Chau and was also due for leave. An English nurse, Joyce Ledger, had returned from leave and would be quite capable of continuing the supervision of the nursing services, where the Chinese staff did most of the actual day to day nursing of the patients. So Kathleen and I decided to go together to Bergen.

We organised an excellent program. When we left Hong Kong in June, 1973, we were clutching a massive bundle of airline tickets, covering about 40 different flights – HK to Bergen via a number of Asian and European stops; then to England, Canada, USA, Hawaii, Fiji, New Zealand and back to Sydney. At the end of that time I would be returning to Hong Kong.

Before we left Hong Kong, we had the job of packing everything up, because it was realised that Hay Ling Chau needed to close. There were now relatively few admissions – happily, we were running out of patients. By the time I left in June 1973, I was able to say that every leprosy patient in Hong Kong who wanted to have reconstructive surgery had been given the opportunity. If they had not had it, it was because they did not want it, or because they were not prepared to co-operate.

Everything had to be packed up and shipped to Australia. In a place like Hong Kong one acquires lovely things. Between us, we had 24 boxes or crates. They did not go till after we had left, but the shipment arrived long before we did, and so my brother Bill and Kathleen's father went down to the wharf to collect them. I had sent Bill the packing list of what was in the crates. Great detailed lists they were! When they arrived at the docks, Customs wanted to know what was in them, as did the quarantine authorities. There are strict rules about bringing plants or animals into Australia for fear of bringing in disease. The Customs people said to my brother, "What's in all these boxes?" and Bill replied, "I do not really know. Here is the list my sister has sent. I know there are quite a lot of gifts that the leprosy patients have made and given to the travellers." At this the fellow looked horrified and just ticked off the list and handed it to Bill and said, "Take it!" We could have smuggled anything in! Bill was amused – as I'd found before, fear of leprosy has its uses. So all our stuff was waiting for us when we got home the following November. My future was still at this stage undecided.

We flew to Bangkok, then on to Nepal, where neither of us had been before. TLM has a hospital at Anandaban, approximately one hour's drive south east of Kathmandu, the capital. We could see the mountains – white shimmering peaks – as we came in through the pass to the Kathmandu valley. Even then smog shrouded the hills – it was bad then but air pollution is much worse today.

Dr Yo Yuasa from Japan met us at the airport. Yo had been one of my students in 1969, and was now working at the Anandaban Hospital, where he assisted Dr John Harris. John had previously worked in Africa, and I had met him in Karigiri, India. He had been superintendent and surgeon at Anandaban for at least five years and he too was going to the Leprosy Congress. Yo was to be Acting Superintendent for the next year until John came back or other arrangements were made.

Yo drove us to the hospital, which is situated behind one of the hills encircling the valley in which Kathmandu stands. When the mission was looking for somewhere to establish a leprosy hospital, the king had insisted that it must not be in the Kathmandu valley itself, because, he said, the god in the shrine on one of the hills, one of the foremost shrines in Nepal, must not be able to "see" the leprosy hospital. Therefore the hospital is situated on the far side of a ridge of hills on the south eastern side of Kathmandu city. The road to the hospital zigzags along the hills and around to the back. If you take an energetic climb to the top of the hill on which the hospital is built, you can see Kathmandu down in the valley below, and, on a good day, a beautiful view of the Himalayan range. So we were able to see the work and renew friendships with Yo.

Once there we met a number of people involved in the leprosy work, one of whom was an expatriate nurse who had been working in leprosy in Nepal for a long time, and who was basically interested in the rehabilitation of leprosy patients. When she met me, she was not sure what she'd struck! We were sitting in the Land Rover when she came up to talk to us and Yo introduced us. He told her that I was a surgeon and we were going to the conference. "Oh," she said exuberantly, "Isn't it good? We now have an artificial leg workshop in Kathmandu valley, so at last we can chop off all those horrible feet that leprosy patients have and give them artificial ones!"

I almost blew my top! What I had been trying to do was to save feet. Given the knowledge of how to look after it, any patient is far, far better off with his own foot than with an artificial leg. As I often have to explain, if you give a patient an artificial leg, first, it is expensive to make at the outset; second, it can quite frequently need repair; third, it is going to need replacement every few years; and fourth, it is very difficult to work, say in rice paddies, with an artificial leg. Think of all that water and mud! There are many other things that rural people in particular cannot do with an artificial leg.

The other problem is that because of their reduced pain perception, friction from the artificial limb is likely to cause leprosy patients to develop ulcers on the stump which may affect the whole leg. We aimed to reconstruct deformed feet to enable patients to wear a shoe. And with good insoles and daily care, they could walk and work without constantly ulcerating their feet. This was, in fact, the subject of my Master's thesis: treating and reconstructing deformed and ulcerated feet, so that the patients did not need to have amputations. And this was what I would talk about in Bergen.

When she was confronted by all this, my new acquaintance had difficulty knowing how to take it! It exploded all that she had come to believe. Yet artificial limbs *were* needed by some – I hope I was not too hard on her! I did visit this limb workshop in the grounds of a big Christian hospital. It was a program for all disabled people in that Hindu country.

In Anandaban John Harris was doing the tendon transfers which played a very big part in preventing ulcers and deformities. But he had not learnt the same type of foot reconstruction as I did because this had not been part of the work at Karigiri. TLM people at Karigiri were only just beginning to implement the same sort of protocols in looking after feet as I had found effective for years in Hong Kong. Over the following years, I was able to persuade the surgeons at Anandaban and other centres in Nepal to update their attitudes so that they also did these reconstructions.

In New Delhi we visited the Leprosy Mission Office where Dr Victor Das was the director of TLM in Southern Asia. At Agra we saw the Taj Mahal – a treat for Kathleen who had not been to India. On then to Pakistan where, in Karachi, I was welcomed as usual at the Marie Adelaide Leprosy Centre. I did some work for a week or so with them.

We proceeded to Teheran in Iran, then to Isfahan in the south. There we were not looking at leprosy work. Kathleen, through her CMS connections, knew the people who were working in the Blind School and we stayed with them in the premises of the Anglican Church. We were able to worship with them on the Sunday morning. With the organist away, I even got the job of playing the organ for the service. In the evening a service was held out in the church garden which was enclosed by a high stone wall. A choir of the girls from the Blind School sang beautifully and a great full moon came up over the stone wall to light the whole scene. It was lovely to be able to share in this ministry in the name of Christ. Blind children in a place like Iran would otherwise have had little chance of education, at least in the 1970s.

We left Teheran on a British Airways flight to Tel Aviv. When we were well aloft, I asked the steward if we would be anywhere near Mt Ararat. "What?" he asked. "Mt Ararat," I said, "You know – where Noah landed the Ark." But he seemed to know nothing of it.

So we left it at that. But about half an hour later he came down and said, "Oh yes, we may be able to see Mt Ararat. It is sometimes visible from the plane, but it will depend on the clouds." There was obviously a lot of cloud, but later he returned to say, "The Captain says that we are quite likely to see Mt Ararat. If you would like to come up to the cockpit, he would be very glad to give you a better view of it." So up we went to the cockpit with the pilot and the co-pilot. The sky still looked densely clouded. But looking through some sort of telescopic instrument one could see a mountain peak emerging through the clouds. He said it was Mt Ararat. Who was I to argue? So I took a photo through the window with my telephoto camera and lens. There was Mt Ararat peeping through the clouds, some 30,000 ft above Turkey! Eventually we swung down towards Israel, getting a good view of the coastline and the stretches of barrenness, the land settlements and the patterns of fields below.

Once through Customs in Tel Aviv, we took a multiple-hire taxi to Jerusalem, where we had arranged to stay at St. George's, the guest house situated amid the buildings of the Anglican Cathedral about a kilometre from the old city's Damascus Gate. During dinner a night or two later, a new couple joined us at the table. The husband was a tall, very distinguished looking man, and his wife, much smaller, was obviously in some discomfort. The story came out that they had just arrived from Tel Aviv where they had been doing some sightseeing. She had slipped on some steps, had hurt both her wrist and her ankle, and was finding it painful to walk. They wondered where they could get medical attention and learned that there was a French hospital nearby where she would be able to be examined and X-rayed. But it was now around 7.30 pm and they wouldn't be able to get attention till the next day. Also the woman was obviously in considerable pain. Kathleen sidled up to them after dinner and volunteered the fact that I was a doctor. We quickly became the first aid station.

Her ankle was very swollen. We bathed it, rubbing it with liniment and immobilising it with a crepe bandage round a splint made of rolled newspaper. Her hand also needed attention. What to do about that? I wanted to bathe that too, but we could not attend to her hand while she had her foot in the bath. In came her husband grinning broadly. He had found a chamber pot in the bedroom cupboard, beside the bed! How about that? So there she was, sitting on the edge of the bath soaking her feet, while her hand was soaking in the chamber pot! Her wrist appeared broken and I suspected that she might have fractured her ankle as well. We wrapped up her wrist in the same way using newspaper as a splint, gave her a couple of painkillers and sent her to bed. In the course of doing all this, we learned who they were. The gentleman was the Bishop of Liverpool, Dr Stuart Blanch, who later became Archbishop of York, and his wife was Brenda.

The next day the bishop took his wife to the French hospital where they X-rayed her and confirmed that she did have a fracture of the wrist. Her foot was not actually fractured, but she would be better off if they put it in a plaster cast, so she could not put her weight on it. Dr Blanch then spent the next ten days taking his wife around Jerusalem in a wheelchair. He commented, "It's not often that I get the chance to push my wife around!" Later we managed to get the cast converted to a walking cast and she was told she would need her wrist in plaster for about eight weeks. They were so grateful, they asked us to come and see them in Liverpool when we arrived in England – which, some time later, we duly did. We stayed with them at Bishopscourt in Liverpool. We were most amused because the guest room literally had episcopal purple sheets on the beds! They had their own private chapel and each night we attended Evensong there. We spent several days with them and visited other people that we knew in that area.

But back to Jerusalem: we had a marvellous time going in and out of the Old City seeing all the usual tourist things. One day we took the train down to Tel Aviv. Another day we went down to Jericho and stopped at the so-called "Inn of the Good Samaritan". A local bus took us to Bethany and we found our way to the church now built at the site of where Lazarus, Martha and Mary were said to have had their home. Nearby is a tomb said to be where Lazarus was laid when Christ called him forth from the dead. We then climbed the Mount of Olives. In our tour group on that occasion there was a clergyman and somebody suggested that he read the appropriate scriptures. Poor guy – he could not even find them! So between us we found and read the story of Christ entering Jerusalem on a donkey, with the people shouting their *Hosannas.*

From the Mount of Olives one can look down on the whole city of Jerusalem spread out below. Some twenty years later, I was able to go up there again and lecture in the Arab medical school that is part of the hospital there. Further down the hill is the Garden of Gethsemane and the Church of All Nations. Here are the olive trees, some of them hundreds of years old. I do not think anybody really knows how old they are. I found it moving to be able to walk among those ancient gnarled trees and sense something of the history and the atmosphere of that place.

After a week or so in Jerusalem, we travelled by bus along the Jordan River to Galilee. We reached Tiberias where we had arranged to stay in the Presbyterian Hostel on the shore of the Sea of Galilee. I took a beautiful photo of sunrise over the lake, which I had printed as a card some years later. We visited a kibbutz, and other spots – Capernaum, Mt Tabor, Nazareth – names and associations well-known and fascinating to Bible readers like ourselves.

Eventually we flew from Tel Aviv to Athens. Soon after we left Athens a terrorist opened fire at the airport. So we were rather glad that we had managed to get through and away.

Then on to Rome, Geneva and Copenhagen. En route, the

hospitality we received would have added up to a colossal amount. I hate to think what our expenses would have been for all our accommodation, if we had not had friends along the way with whom we could stay and just help by contributing to the costs.

17

Round the World – 2

Then came Norway. We flew into Oslo and stayed for a day or two in a Christian hostel as tourists, before travelling to Bergen to take part in the huge Leprosy Conference. There were probably a thousand delegates; some were accompanying spouses but everybody had an interest in leprosy.

The conference was judged a great success. It included an ecumenical service in four languages in the chapel of the original Hansen Hospital, the old hospital for leprosy patients in Norway. The chapel had old-fashioned box pews, not intended to hold many people. A lot were jammed in that night. The Holy Table I will always remember, because there were two figurines on that table, labelled *Love* and *Faith.*

Of course, we usually think of the trilogy *Faith, Hope* and *Love.* Significantly *Hope* was missing. Carved in a sign over one leprosy hospital in South America was the quotation from Dante's vision of Hell – *"Abandon hope all ye that enter here."* In Hansen's day too, there was no hope of a cure for leprosy, for either the disease or the deformities. In many countries it is still considered a curse of the gods for misconduct in this life or in a previous existence.

Many still believe that all those who get leprosy will eventually become deformed and disabled. They do not realize that in most people it is self-curing, leaving them without any obvious signs of the disease. But in those days in Norway, people once admitted to that hospital had to accept a life sentence.

Norway in the nineteenth century had no means other than isolation to stop the spread of the disease. It was not realized, as we know today, that it is probably mostly spread by coughing and sneezing. When we were in Bergen in 1973 Norway still had about twenty people who had the disease.

I say "had the disease" but unfortunately that statement has officially altered its connotation in recent decades. In 1973, we still kept cumulative records, and every patient who was ever diagnosed as having leprosy was maintained on the record until such time as they died. This was logical because of the belief that its effects would be life-long. In 1973 we still spoke of the fact that there were probably 15 million people in the world with leprosy, of whom probably one in five (20%), were deformed or disabled to some degree. By that I mean having an obvious deformity or disability, a paralysis or loss of pain perception – I do not mean just having skin patches.

In the 1940s the effective treatment, dapsone was found to control the disease, kill the germs and stop them from multiplying. This drug brought a completely new outlook on leprosy. Patients who had the disease could be rendered non-infectious – they would not pass the disease on to other people and were less likely to develop disability. However, then the World Health Organization aimed to remove leprosy as a public health problem; by this they meant that they would reduce the chance of people contracting leprosy when living in the community. They stated that they would do this by the year 2005. (Originally they said 2000 – now they say 2010!)

Part of their program has been to redefine leprosy, so that to be registered as a leprosy patient, a person must have the lesions of leprosy and be receiving effective anti-leprosy medication. WHO recognized that they do not now need life-long treatment, and recommends much shorter duration of specific drugs. Once the drugs cease, the patient is removed from the list of those with leprosy. Those of us with many years of experience are very fearful that these shortened courses of medication are going to result in many relapses. We are already seeing too many occur.

Not everybody agrees with the WHO, but that is now the

standard definition. The statistics that are now produced are really statistics of the number of leprosy patients who are currently on treatment. The standard fails to take into account the number that cease treatment too soon; nor does it take into account the millions who have a deformity and a disfigurement of body or mind, perhaps socially, because at some stage in the past they have had leprosy.

In the rural villages of third world countries, people are afraid of leprosy and hate it very strongly. Many countries do not want to notify that they have a high incidence of leprosy. That is something of which they are ashamed.

The new statistics, as given out today in the early twenty-first century, make it look as though leprosy is nearly eliminated. I wish that was so. I am afraid that it is not. I am afraid that the politics, the necessity of watching the amount of money that is spent on treatment of this chronic disease, has resulted in many patients stopping treatment too soon.

I am also afraid that this may well mean that in years to come – even up to 30 – we will have a sudden increase in the number of people with leprosy. Who knows? What we do know is that the leprosy germ is a very clever organism. It can become resistant to the drugs that we have to treat it and so we usually give two or three different drugs at the same time to minimise that chance of resistance. It can also lie dormant in the body for many years. We call these "persister bacilli", ones that persist in the patient's body in spite of good medication. It appears that the bacilli can survive tucked away in nerves and muscles, out of reach of antibiotics. Once treatment is discontinued the bacteria emerge and start to multiply again.

A lot of this was discussed at Bergen. What could or should we do about it? How were we to treat patients more effectively, and more cost effectively? How could these special drugs that we now have be delivered to the patients who needed them? – and how were they to be paid for? The patients certainly could not afford these drugs. Who was going to provide the funds for the paramedicals and others to go tramping the hills of countries like Nepal and Pakistan, finding the patients who needed the treatment? This was all part of what that conference was about.

At that conference I chaired the session on Rehabilitation Surgery. What we discussed was basically simple material: how to diagnose and treat disabilities of various types. It was now 20 to 25 years since Paul Brand realised that a lot could be done surgically to help leprosy patients. Most leprosy patients have one or more of only five or six physical deformities. There are routine procedures to help them. Paul Brand's work showed us that, in many instances, what he recommended was certainly the best procedure available, and applicable in many other diseases and conditions. Each of the dozens of other procedures has its own problems. One cannot just deal with patients in an assembly line fashion, shuffling them through and doing them all the same way. Each patient must be treated as an individual. What are we going to do for this particular person? How are we going to help this unique person?

At the Bergen Conference the same factors showed up again. It has never ceased to amaze me that I, never an academic achiever, now found myself in positions of medical and surgical influence. I suppose I do have persistence and determination. Having got my teeth into the problems of reconstructive surgery, I hung on. So I found myself in the chair of the rehabilitation section, guiding others in the presentation of their topics and chairing the discussion from the whole body of experts gathered in that hall at that time.

Kath and I had decided that we could not leave Norway after the conference without seeing something of the country. Four of us arranged to go on a trip to Balestrand. It was on a fjord, some way north of Bergen – a place of beautiful tranquillity, mountains coming down into the sea and snow-capped hills, cold and crisp. It was so good to get away for a few days and relax after all the bustle of the conference.

Next stop was London. There we stayed in the flat on the top story of the TLM offices in a renovated heritage house in Portland Place, near the BBC studios and All Souls, Langham Place, a favourite church. A beautiful sweeping staircase led from the front door up to the next level where there were some meeting rooms. On the third floor were the offices and above that two small flats: one for the caretaker, the other with guest rooms for people like us. Early each morning we saw the horses trot out of Buckingham Palace to exercise in Hyde Park – a delight to Kathleen who loves horses.

It was an excellent place, right in the heart of London, to have as a base. I spoke at some TLM meetings – and by that time, I had come to realize that God's plan for me was to travel and to teach. Staying there gave me an excellent opportunity to get to know some of the London staff. One was Eddie Askew, who for many years, was the International Director of The Leprosy Mission. Eddie was also a fine artist and a writer of many devotional books which have become popular. I have used extracts from them in my circular letters and have given them away as gifts.

I had long talks with Eddie about future plans and staff. One concern was that the staff were constantly changing. Keen young workers would offer to the Mission and we would send them out, train them to become useful – and then they would come home on leave and decide not to return. So we would need to find and train someone else. Other missions and humanitarian organizations experienced the same high turnover problem. We talked about what we could do to encourage young people, with a heart for serving others, to take up leprosy work in particular, and missionary work in general, as a lifetime job.

In medicine particularly, people need to get the right training and develop links early, or they may miss out on vital career opportunities. Young doctors may fear never being able achieve career goals. Certainly that is what the world says, but since I committed my life to missionary work, because I believed that was God's will for me, I have found that he has gone ahead of me and has prepared each new step. I have also seen many of my colleagues, who have given a large part of their active life to helping in Third World countries, face the inevitable question, on arrival home, "What are you going to do now? How are you going to find a job?" Yet often that question has been answered absolutely marvellously.

One young surgeon, for example, worked as a professor in a hospital in Asia as part of his missionary job. He had to return to Australia because of family illness, yet within a year he was offered another professorship, in Australia this time. God trains those who want to work for him, so that they are ready for the job that he has planned for them. He does not desert those who really seek to serve him. There is an old statement: "God does not choose those who are fit for the task. He fits those who are prepared to follow where he leads."

Eddie Askew and I discussed my future. I was by now a long-term member of the mission. It was 14 years since I had started in Hong Kong even though I only went there on a temporary basis initially. I now had a lot of hands-on experience. I had worked in a number of different countries. I was beginning to understand something of the problems of the different cultures and their customs and beliefs and how this affected what we could do for their people. I also appreciated the problem that students and trainees in leprosy were often sent to a place of excellence to work and learn, and then, when they returned to their medical centre, were not allowed to do what they had been taught. Their superiors' attitude blocked and frustrated the more highly trained student: "Oh, we have always done it this way – there is no need to change!"

Hence it was obvious to me, and it also became obvious to TLM, that a better and more cost-effective way to produce good results was for a teacher to go and teach regularly in an institution. If doctors from that institution were given the same amount of cash to go and study somewhere else, they would be studying and learning to do things they might never encounter; learning to use equipment that could never be afforded; and not be learning how to deal with the actual problems they encountered daily. So I was ready with these thoughts for discussions regarding my future and what I was to do. "I will go anywhere – anywhere there is a need for training and teaching and surgery to benefit people with leprosy." That is basically what I told Eddie Askew. He certainly appreciated the ideas I had for an itinerant ministry, travelling and teaching, and he supported me wholeheartedly. And that became the story of the next fifteen years of my life and beyond. In fact we devised a plan whereby I would be directly under him as International Director and not under one of the regional directors. As I would be working all over the world, when a request came for me to visit a certain country, I merely had to refer it to Eddie.

When I was speaking at meetings, I took this as my theme. In Isaiah 54, God says to Israel:

"Enlarge the place of your tent and let the curtains of your habitations be stretched out. Hold not back. Lengthen your cords, and strengthen your stakes, for you will spread abroad to the right and to the left."

I accepted that this was God's commission to me – that he was leading me to go and 'spread abroad' and to teach methods of treating leprosy that were not yet adopted in many areas, so that many more people could benefit from the methods and treatments that we were now able to use.

It has been fascinating since 1973 actually to see this come to fruition, because I have been enabled to work in so many countries, helping leprosy patients. But I and my colleagues are also missionaries – literally 'sent ones' – obeying Jesus' command to share the gospel by word and deed, showing forth the love of God. It's true that in many of the countries where I have worked I do not speak the local language, but, by my actions and care, I hope that I show the love of God to those who are in need. In fact I've been told of patients saying, "We wish she could speak our language – we know she loves us."

I hear it again and again, even now, that people who come to me with problems due to nerve damage have been brushed aside by others with the comment, "Ah well, you cannot expect that to get better – you have just got to learn to live with it!" Well, do you? Is that what God really wants for them? He has given us the ability, not to cure everyone, by any means, but certainly to help make life more livable for a large number of people with deformities and disabilities. On that trip over thirty years ago, I felt that this was my challenge. I did not know how it was going to work or what I was going to do, but I was certain that my job in the future was certainly not to be an administrator. I had seen too many good clinicians end up behind a desk pushing a pen, hardly ever able to see and treat a patient in the flesh.

But our time in England was not just meetings – it was a delightful chance for sightseeing. We were able to rent a car, get around and see various friends in Oxford and southern England and Scotland, and enjoy London too.

From London we boarded a jumbo jet for the trip across the Atlantic. As we were travelling west, we landed in Toronto apparently several hours before we left England. 10 pm Toronto time was for us about 2 am. Our very pleasant and generous Canadian hosts took us home, offered us a meal and wanted to sit and talk. It was all we could do to keep awake! Over the next few days, there were a number of TLM meetings to speak at and we also threw in some sightseeing, including the Niagara Falls.

The next major stop was at the Public Health Service Hospital at Carville, Louisiana, the official US Government Leprosy Institution where Dr Paul Brand was then a staff member. The long-established hospital – closed in 1998 after 104 years – was on the banks of the Mississippi 70 miles north of New Orleans. Initially it was run by Roman Catholic nuns. By the seventies there were very few nuns amongst the staff. We shared the morning service in the chapel where Margaret Brand sang in the choir. We stayed in the staff quarters but we spent a lot of time with the Brands, seeing around the hospital which had all the "mod cons" the patients could ask for. It was easy to see why they did not want to be discharged!

I was very interested in Paul's research into the function of the individual muscles of the arm, which became the basis for a major book on the mechanics of the hand that he published. He also did a lot of work on pressure in hands and feet and on the part played in ulcer formation by pressure during everyday activities, including research into devices to protect hands and feet during use.

We saw the armadillos living in Carville housed securely in pens with concrete walls and floors, because of their tunnelling skill. They were used in research into the leprosy organism as they are one of the few animals in which the leprosy bacilli can be easily cultivated.

Then it was on to Los Angeles as the guests of Len Marmour, who had worked as an orthopaedic surgeon in Hong Kong. He specialized in knee replacements and the car he lent us had an easily recognised number plate – *KNEE.*

From there we flew to Vancouver. Here again, the local TLM secretary met us and accommodated us in his home. He had a number of church services lined up for us. On the Sunday, he made use of both of us – Kathleen spoke to the Sunday School while I spoke in the main church. He took us then to a restaurant at which, on a Sunday at lunchtime, the preacher dines free. Since he was an ordained minister, and as I was the preacher at the main church that morning, and Kathleen had been the preacher at the Sunday school, the only one who had to pay was his wife!

After our time in North America we flew to Hawaii. Though I was a veteran traveller in Asian countries, in America I was a new and green tourist, and it was fascinating to me that all these places I'd heard and read about were becoming a reality. The tour meant pleasure mixed with work. Hawaii, of course, was where the famous Father Damien had worked back in 1873. So that date kept cropping up. In 1873 in Norway, Hansen discovered the leprosy bacillus. In that same year Father Damien went to work at Molokai. And it was in 1873 that The Leprosy Mission really started. The pioneer missionary, Dr Wellesley Bailey, was speaking at a church meeting in Dublin, Ireland, about the leprosy patients he had been helping in India. Two of the ladies present, the Misses Pim, decided to raise funds to help. Within a few years they had raised so much money that they had to find more mission groups to use the funds. Thus the specialist Mission to Lepers was founded. In that one year God brought about all three momentous events in different parts of the world in which people began to deal with the scourge of leprosy in a serious, systematic way – medically, socially and spiritually.

18

Round the World – 3

In Hawaii we settled ourselves in one of the many hotels. It served buffet type meals with a notice: "Take what you can eat – but eat what you take!" Our philosophy exactly!

We took the opportunity of a visit to the island of Molokai, the site of the leprosarium where Father Damien had lived and worked. Damien was a Belgian priest who felt called to serve the leprosy patients of Hawaii. He lived with them on the island of Molokai where they were confined. Once a patient was admitted, he expected never to leave. So Father Damien was signing himself in for a lifetime of segregation. As the stories tell it, one day in about 1885 he spilled boiling water on his foot and realised that it was anaesthetic – that he also had leprosy and that he would never leave Molokai and his beloved patients.

Damien worked there until his death in 1889. A chapel stands in his memory on the Kalapapa Peninsula which projects to the north of the island. For many years the official government hospital was on Molokai and everybody with leprosy was sent there for treatment. Most of the patients lived in family units in small cottages scattered around the island. The main part of the island was an area of higher ground, where people lived who were not patients, but ordinary healthy people who made a living by buying and selling goods to the leprosy settlement.

We took a plane to Molokai and were taken on a guided tour of the leprosy colony. Not many patients lived there then, though there were still a number of elderly and disabled people. We learned that now there was another leprosy treatment area in Hawaii and that most people were treated as outpatients. I am glad I visited Kalapapa.

I had read about it and seen old films and it helped me to appreciate the deep, almost superstitious, fear held then for leprosy. Yet one is no more likely to catch leprosy and develop leprosy than any other infectious disease – and at least it is now treatable.

We flew on to Fiji. In Suva we stayed at the Anglican Guest House where lovely local girls looked after us. We explored the place a bit, being scheduled to be there only for a few days.

On the afternoon of the last full day, Kathleen decided that she would like to get a photograph of the girls with hibiscus flowers in their hair, dressed in their brightly coloured sarongs. So outside the guest house there were was much laughter and carrying on as she got them lined up. Kath was just ready to take a photo when a dog rushed out from the house next door, latched on to her leg and took a bite of it. It was a big bite and left a whole line of tooth marks and torn muscles.

So I was on medical duty! I usually travel with a bit of a medical kit, but I certainly did not have enough for that! I put a rough bandage around it and we took ourselves by taxi to the local public hospital. A young Fijian doctor was on duty. He was sitting in casualty with a long line of patients waiting to see him, when in came these two foreign women, one pushing the other in a wheelchair. They readily provided a table and space for me to deal with the emergency myself. I used a local anaesthetic and cleaned and stitched Kath's leg and gave her a tetanus shot. It was quite a nasty gash. I got antibiotics, crepe bandages and various odds and ends from the pharmacy before we headed back to our accommodation, where we worked out a way of keeping the leg elevated for the night.

The following day we were going to New Zealand. I phoned our hosts to let them know what had happened and asked them please to be ready with a pair of crutches at the airport. It was fun and games getting Kath on and off planes. At Nadi, one of the Fijians met us with a wheelchair and pushed us around the airport to do all that was necessary before we were to catch the flight to Auckland. Boarding required us to climb a long flight of steps. I plodded up with all our hand luggage while the Fijian who had been pushing the wheelchair just picked Kath up in his arms and carried her up – no problem whatsoever! I was too slow to get the camera out for a photo!

At Auckland they brought her down in the food lift, and a Maori was waiting for us with a wheelchair. He immediately escorted us through the airport, and that was one of the quickest arrivals and immigrations we have ever done! Bob Alcorn, the local TLM director, was waiting in his car with a pair of crutches.

We stayed at the home of the Rev David Stewart, who had gone through university with my brother. He had been the headmaster of the school at Darjeeling where I had visited in 1963. We had many TLM meetings to take in New Zealand. In fact we were there for about a month and I think I spoke at about 40 meetings.

One of the early ones was at a local Anglican church. We arrived mid-week and David Stewart said with a big grin, "Well, Father John would like to come and see you. When he booked you to speak at his service, he thought you were Dr Graham Warren – he did not realise you wore skirts! He wants to check you out to see whether he thinks you are suitable for speaking at his church!" So, in due course, Father John arrived.

Many university students attended that Sunday evening healing service, with prayer on request. I decided then to speak about Jesus healing the man at the pool of Bethesda. (John 5) "Do you want to be healed?" Jesus asked. An excellent question! For many people who come to me, leprosy patients and others, yes, they would love to be healed as long as it can happen instantly, and they do not have to work at it!

But in healing services, some may seek prayer for healing who do not really want to get better. Part of their identity lies in having something wrong with them. So in my address I aimed a double barrelled shotgun at both situations. There was much that God could do to heal them if they truly wanted it. But if they wanted to hang on to their 'deformities', their multiple problems, well, not even God could help them. So – did they want to be healed?

I felt it was an excellent service and a lot of people commented on it. Afterwards, supper was served down in the crypt, and then I presented a half an hour of slides on the actual leprosy work that I was doing. Father John said that a good number of people came up and thanked him afterwards for the whole evening.

I was able to go to the Middlemoor Hospital where leprosy patients are treated, and I met various people who were involved with leprosy, although in New Zealand there are not many with the disease. We travelled to Rotorua to see the usual tourist attractions. Then it was south by train to Wellington, where again we had various meetings, before flying across to Blenheim on the south island and eventually to Dunedin where I was able to lecture at the university. One of their hand surgeons had done some surgery with me in Hong Kong and wanted me to talk to the students about leprosy.

I was also privileged to preach in the First Presbyterian Church because the Moderator realised that I had worked with the Presbyterians in Korea. In Queenstown we had a couple of days "off duty". We arrived on the day that Princess Anne was to be married and watched the telecast of the wedding ceremony that night. The next day we went up a mountain on a ski lift where we enjoyed the snow and the views.

At Christchurch Cathedral we were part of a group of speakers at a well attended inter-mission gathering for CMS, OMF and TLM. One of the subjects discussed was leprosy work in Africa because CMS has quite a lot of people there. I had not actually been to Africa at that stage.

We returned to the North Island and eventually back to Sydney. By this time, Kath's leg had healed well. She will have a scar on her leg to the end of her days – you can see where the muscle was damaged but it works all right and that is the main thing.

We arrived home in late November 1973, ready to organise for Christmas and the summer conventions and house-parties. I was due for furlough, and, in theory, would be on leave until the middle of 1974, when I would return to Hong Kong or some other part of Asia. We had not yet determined where I would be working. Nor did we know then the actual date on which Hay Ling Chau would be closed.

For both of us it had been a marvellous trip. It had enabled us to see the variations of leprosy work in many countries of the world. We had met in their home territories lots of people with whom we had worked overseas, and had met supporters and made many new friends. And believe it or not, we had had a thoroughly good break!

This trip marked the end of the first fifteen years of my overseas service. It so happens that my life seems to fall neatly into fifteen-year segments. Now I was ready for the next step.

19

WIDER RECOGNITION: AUSTRALIA

I spent the first half of 1974 in Australia, mainly doing Leprosy Mission deputation and commencing what could be described as my medical consultation program. Previously I had done very little surgery in Australia, but in 1974 there were those who realised that surgically I was doing something worthwhile. I had been nominated for a Fellowship of the Royal Australasian College of Surgeons, and that helped spread word that my work was valuable. So, I received a number of requests for consultation and to do surgery for patients in Australia.

One of these came for a girl, aged about 19, who had been in a horrific car accident some years earlier – a head-on collision when she and a group of young people were driving home from church. She had suffered head injuries and various fractures, including a badly fractured leg which had left her with a foot-drop.

An orthopaedic surgeon was consulted to straighten the badly deformed toes on the affected foot. This surgeon knew my work and asked me to see her. Then together we did the surgery, straightened her toes, and changed the tendons around so that she could lift her foot properly when she walked. This gave her the chance of walking normally, like any other young person. The whole project was rather amusing. We had a long talk beforehand as to what I could and could not do. I said that after surgery, yes, she would be able to lift her foot a certain way, but she wouldn't have a full, normal range of movement. So she really needed to tell me whether she preferred to be able to wear high heels or to be able to walk barefoot, or to wear sports-type shoes.

She decided high heels were not a priority. So that is what we did for her, and I can still visualise the morning in Sydney Hospital when we allowed her to walk without appliances for the first time. She had been having intensive physiotherapy and had learnt how to use the transferred muscle. At first she had needed to walk stiff-legged. The day arrived when I was prepared to let her try to walk normally. Her father had brought her in and I told her to walk the length of the corridor, allowing her knees to bend. Her father nearly disintegrated into tears.

He said, "Why on earth did not somebody do this for her years ago?" Here was a girl whose whole gait – and therefore her life – had been transformed. She was now able to walk basically normally wearing a normal shoe. It was simply that that particular operation, while commonplace to me, was a rarity here in Australia.

Well, they were thrilled. However, there was a hitch. Looking rather shame-faced, she said, "I am being a bridesmaid in a few weeks' time, and we are all wearing stilt heels!" And I had carefully operated so she could walk with low heels! But fortunately the hospital had a shoemaker who could help. He built up the soles of the shoes she wanted to wear with cork so her feet were level as if in flat shoes, but she looked as though she had high heels.

I saw her next about three years later; by which time she had married. She had worn high heels so much that her foot was down in a position that enabled her to do that. Now flat shoes may have been a difficulty, but this did not matter. She'd adapted. Her foot no longer caused her any major problems and most people did not even realize it had been damaged.

Ever since that time I have been asked to do work like this whenever I am back in Australia. In 1974 people discovered that I had done a lot of tendon work, transferring the tendons to give better function in hands and feet, and, to a lesser extent, in the face. So the specialists in these different fields were more than happy to have me working with them so that I could teach them what I knew.

That was the beginning of a program that I had never dreamt I would get involved in, but which has gone on expanding over the following thirty years.

At the same time, I was speaking to many TLM and church groups, gaining financial and prayer support and explaining the work we were doing. I was also contacting various other countries in the process of deciding what I was going to do next. It was by then generally known that Hay Ling Chau would close in January 1975 – so I would not be going back there long term. I would just call in and do what surgery was needed at the end of 1974. But where next? There were numerous suggestions and invitations. Could I come to this centre, to help and to teach? Could I relieve so and so at such and such a hospital? We weighed up all these pros and cons.

I was asked to become the superintendent of another TLM hospital, with the promise, the "carrot" – "Oh, you could still go off and teach sometimes!" But I knew that being superintendent of a whole hospital would allow little time for me to go off and teach elsewhere. I had glimpsed that there was more than enough work to keep me going full time in a roving advisory and teaching role – and this was what I knew I could most usefully do. God had given me the vision of travelling and teaching as I had discussed with Eddie Askew in London.

So I turned that one down, together with other similar offers.

By mid-year it was time for me to head off on the program that we had devised. It started with my first visit to Perth.

I stayed with a loyal TLM supporter, and was invited to lecture at a medical college and to visit the rehabilitation centre, the Charles Gardiner Centre, where George Bedbrook (by that time Sir George) had done his work. It was George who had come through Hong Kong at the end of 1964 and suggested that I could do bone surgery. So it was quite a thrill to go and see his patients, and even more to be asked to attend one of the early morning doctors' discussion groups. Here we looked at a child born with spina bifida (a congenital condition where the base of the spine hasn't developed normally, usually resulting in some abnormality of the feet). This particular child's feet did not look too bad and he could walk, but he had ulcers which just wouldn't heal. Of course, this was exactly the work I had been doing; these were neuropathic ulcers due to lack of proper nerve sensation in the feet, which I knew would heal if adequately rested. So I was able to share that information. Again our work in leprosy came to be of benefit to people in the developed world.

That flight to Perth was delayed leaving Sydney and we were given a hotel room overnight. I woke feeling absolutely lousy as I was coming down with flu. A particularly vicious virus was around that year and it targeted my laryngeal nerve. For months, all through that trip, I was coping with a hoarse, croaking voice which I could not rest because I had talks and lectures to give. I spoke at some medical and mission meetings in Perth and then flew north up the coast to Darwin.

There I was met by Dr John Hargrave, who was in charge of the leprosy program for the Northern Territory Government. In India in the 1960s, he'd learnt about reconstructive surgery and rehabilitation, which had not up to that time been implemented in Australia. En route there he had called into Hong Kong. I remembered sitting on the veranda of our house on the island with John, talking about surgery. He then scrubbed in with me for a couple of hand operations. So I probably taught John his first leprosy operations. On this trip I was able to do some surgery with him in the Darwin Base Hospital.

He went on to do many of these operations, not only in North Australia but also in West Timor, where he visited to help with the leprosy and other rehabilitation programs. John retired a couple of years after I did. He had made a name for himself with the aboriginal leprosy programs, and succeeded in changing the whole attitude of people in the Northern Territory to leprosy.

Leprosy was brought into Australia by the indentured Chinese labourers in the 1880/90s, and, in the Territory, it rapidly entered the indigenous communities. Aborigines had no fear of this new and unknown disease. So when they developed skin patches, they ignored them. They did not hurt or itch and not a great many people were affected – usually less than 5% of any population will ever develop leprosy – but even so an increasing number of people in the aboriginal settlements developed deformities and disabilities.

In aboriginal culture people are bound spiritually to their own place – to their birthplace, to their forebears and to the spirits of the land. For an aboriginal person to leave his own territory can be a major problem. When the white man tried to take away people with leprosy and put them into hospital in Darwin, they objected. This reached its peak in the 1920/30s, for if they were taken away, they never came back. So those with leprosy did their best to hide from visiting medical officers. They certainly did not volunteer to be treated.

John changed and modernised the whole program. He arranged for the leprosy patients to be seen in their own settlements, camps and reserves, and to be treated by the nurses responsible for the welfare and the health clinics in those areas. As a result, more of the patients who had early signs of leprosy would come for treatment, because now they knew they did not have to go to Darwin. They knew that they would not be taken away from their own tribal area.

When it came to surgery, John soon made it well known that although, they would have to come to Darwin for their operations, once the surgery was over, they could return to their own community in a better physical state and be better able to care for themselves.

In these ways John Hargrave altered the whole picture of leprosy in North Australia. I was privileged to have John show me his work.

I was thrilled much later, in 1999, to share with John an inaugural award given by the Royal Australasian College of Surgeons "For a Lifetime of Surgery." (See chapter 37)

John took me out to some of the aboriginal settlements, including Oenpelli, a CMS mission in Arnhem Land. I accompanied the doctor in an aerial ambulance on one of his regular trips, and also flew over to Groote Eylandt where my parents had worked and where my brother David was born. From Darwin I headed back to Hong Kong via Singapore and Kuala Lumpur. Although Hay Ling Chau was now winding down, there were a number of patients needing reconstructive surgery, so I had a surgical spree in Hong Kong doing that work.

On that particular trip, I ended up with a very bad ear infection. All my life I have had problems with my ears when flying, but that was the worst episode, developing after yet another small plane flight. I had ruptured my left eardrum, probably because of that bout of influenza I'd had in Perth. I was living on antibiotics and other medication trying to get better.

From Hong Kong, with my bottles of pills, I flew to Taiwan, a place I had visited often. On this longer trip I did my usual round of the island. Chapter 20 tells more about this visit and the work in Taiwan.

Then I returned to Hong Kong for the final Open Day of the institution at the end of 1974. By the time it actually closed in January 1975, I was in Pakistan.

20

Taiwan through the years

I first went to the Republic of China (Taiwan) in 1960, where, as mentioned in chapter 10, I met Ruth Lin. She spoke a Chinese dialect and ran a leprosy clinic on the west coast at Tainan. Further south, in the city of Kaohsiung, a residential leprosy clinic for about 20/30 patients was established, managed by a Presbyterian pastor, the Rev John, who was also a laboratory technician. Doctors came from the Kaohsiung Medical College to observe, to teach leprosy to the students and to help with the treatment of the patients.

Further east is a Christian hospital at Pingdung, and another small residential leprosy hospital. In each case, the leprosy hospital or clinic is situated well away from the main hospital, because of the fear of leprosy amongst the Chinese. The dread of leprosy had been passed on down through the years and had caused tragic attitudes. For instance, if a dermatologist was known to treat leprosy in his skin clinic, he was likely to find that he would have no other patients, because they were afraid that they might sit next to a leprosy patient and catch the disease themselves.

There were lots of these notions about leprosy. This fear alters people's judgements. In medicine we always say that "You only recognise what you want to recognise – you only see what you look for". I often hear of patients being wrongly diagnosed in ordinary clinics. Probably the doctors did not want to diagnose leprosy because they knew that the patients did not want to have it! So if they had symptoms that might be due to leprosy, but could also be due to other diseases, if at all possible they would be diagnosed and treated for the other diseases. We still find that even in Australia. A patient had been treated in a major teaching hospital for several years for sciatica, although the symptoms he had in his leg did not really match that diagnosis. It was only after several years of deterioration that it was realised that he actually had leprosy!

In the far south of Taiwan is Hengchun, with another Christian hospital and leprosy clinic. On that trip in 1974, I was very gratified because there were by then a number of doctors who were interested in leprosy and were seriously getting involved in the program. But few were doing reconstructive surgery, nor did there seem to be much demand for it – probably because the patients did not realise what could be done, and so they just put up with their deformities.

Previously I had done surgery at the Changhua Christian Hospital on the west coast. The leprosy clinic there was run by a Danish nurse, Gerda, another who had worked in China. She spoke Mandarin and had done a marvellous job in leprosy treatment for years. Patients who were diagnosed with leprosy at the big Changhua hospital were sent out to Gerda's clinic – really a small hospital. Gerda was a wonderful nurse – a very capable woman. She was more than happy to have me visiting, teaching her and helping with problem patients. We were able to operate on a number of patients from her clinic. For their surgery they were admitted to the Changhua hospital in the morning and taken back to her clinic in the evening where she would look after them.

I remember one episode with horror. There was an elderly woman who had a total facial paralysis. She could not close her lips at all and her eyes were permanently open; her appearance was so grotesque it made her almost an outcast. So we agreed to do some reconstructive surgery for her to enable her to close her eyes and to correct some of her other problems.

We took this elderly lady – we will call her Sui-an – to the operation room and had a great discussion beforehand about her artificial teeth. She wanted to be able to wear her teeth after the surgery. If we did not have them in when we were operating, we wouldn't know how to shape her mouth as we repaired it. So we left the false teeth in place while we were operating. Then she was bandaged up and sent back to the clinic, with the teeth still in place.

Sui-an's hands and feet were also badly affected; in fact, she virtually had no fingers. But we had decided to do the face first. But Sui-an did not really understand what had been done for her and what her own part had to be.

On the third morning when I went to see Sui-an, I discovered that during the night she had decided that she wanted the false teeth out. How she removed them I do not know. She had no fingers on her hand and I had fashioned a tendon 'sling' of skin to lift her bottom lip into position. But out they came. In so doing, she broke the newly attached tendon on one side. Despite all this, although the final result was far from what I hoped to have achieved, she was certainly vastly improved in appearance – and she was satisfied.

Our patients were often simple peasant folk and it was very hard to make them understand what we were doing and why. You can try to explain the process but when they wake up from the anaesthetic and find, say, they have an arm in plaster, they do not realise why they needed to have it in a certain position. We needed to put on plaster strong enough not to be broken and to hold the repaired tissues protected so healing could occur.

Just down the road from Gerda's clinic, there was a Roman Catholic rehabilitation clinic run by a lovely sister – Sr Antonio, a doctor from the United States. Here they did a lot for people with disabilities from any cause – particularly poliomyelitis. Sr Antonio was a very enthusiastic helper of Gerda in arranging for the rehabilitation of patients, particularly those with foot problems.

At Changhua I was able to work with an American doctor, Dr Joe Wilkerson. He was officially a general surgeon, and, in those days, they were literally 'general' – called upon to do anything. He was no exception. On a number of occasions he had patients with very interesting problems for me to discuss with him and sometimes I operated on them.

One young girl had cerebral palsy and as a result her right arm was affected. The wrist was permanently bent down so that she was unable to use her hand properly. I was able to move some of the muscles on her arm in exactly the same way as I do for leprosy, so that the muscle which bent her wrist down into flexion, reversed its action so that it could pull her wrist up into extension. We were thus able to give this child a functional grip. It made so much difference to her because then she was able to hold a pencil at school and to write and to do all sorts of things previously difficult or impossible.

Another patient, a young man of twenty, had been severely burnt, particularly on one leg. There were lots of raw areas where the tissue would not heal over. The tissues had begun to heal in some places but the wounds kept breaking down as he used his leg. Dr Joe asked me if I could do anything for him. So I told him about a relatively simple procedure, whereby we removed all the poor quality scar tissue and treated the healthier tissue beneath it so that it would take a new skin graft. We wrapped the leg in bandages left it for a week for healing to commence, and then covered it with the skin graft that had been kept in the fridge. Then we carefully wrapped it up again and left it to heal. In that first operation we got about eighty to ninety percent of the leg covered with new skin and getting the rest of it healed was then a small job. Dr Joe was very pleased to have learnt that trick. This method was much simpler than the 'flap skin grafts' which were commonly used at that time. Dr Joe had a real interest in his patients and their welfare. One never knew what one might see in his clinics. It was wonderfully rewarding to work with him because I had the opportunity of honing skills in areas which I normally would not have encountered.

In Taipei itself, I used to do a leprosy clinic at the big Christian hospital, the Mackay Memorial Hospital. Later a Chinese dermatologist looked after those leprosy patients. Meanwhile the Government Leprosy Hospital, where I had first gone for just for a day in 1960, was still as busy as ever. Many who lived in that hospital did not really need to be inpatients, but because of the stigma of leprosy in the Chinese community as a whole, they preferred to stay there.

Every time I visited Taiwan I went to that hospital. One patient was said to have a lepra reaction, but I discovered that it was not that at all. It was relapse. He had started treatment years before and as soon as he thought he was getting better, he'd stopped his medication and disappeared. Eventually he came back with more symptoms. He was put back on the same treatment but again stopped too early and vanished. So here he was for the third time. When you looked at his back, you could see that there were three concentric rings where the leprosy lesion had kept recurring just because he wouldn't take his medication for long enough. So this was a very important point to try and get through to the patients and to the staff. You have to go on treating leprosy until you have got rid of all the bacteria that are present in those lesions.

In 1974 when I visited the clinic, I was asked to see another patient who looked as though he had an acute lepra reaction of the antibody antigen type. (See chapter 14) He was covered with little red spots. The doctor was querying the fact that they were not responding to the steroid treatment he was giving. When I had a look at him, I said, "Yes, but that is not reaction – those are new leprosy lesions. This man has relapsed."

"Oh no, he hasn't, we have looked for bacteria and he hasn't got any", the doctor replied.

I said, "I think he has bacteria".

"Oh, no, no – the lab. technician says they cannot find any."

"All right then, I want a smear taken now, and when the lab. technician has stained it, I will go and have a look at it myself under the microscope," I responded.

So I took the smear and gave it to the technician to stain and asked him to call me when it was ready. In due course he called me and said that there were no leprosy bacilli present.

I put the slide under the microscope myself – and found it was absolutely teaming with bacilli. Then we discovered that this particular technician was only very briefly and casually examining these slides. We also discovered afterwards that a lot of the patients actually bribed him to say that they had no bacteria in their smears, because they did not want to have these bacteria signifying active leprosy. It was also a good lesson for the doctors that they should every now and then look at the microscope smears for themselves, to make sure that they have been properly taken and examined.

It was therefore a very valuable morning, a time when we discovered that many patients were being under-treated because of the customs and the culture of that particular area.

Built on a hillside outside Taipei, Taiwan's capital, there was another leprosy hospital, which was run by an order of German Lutheran sisters. I used to stay with them in their home and share in the work of the centre. They did not normally have surgery at that centre, but occasionally we did some operations in the outpatients' clinic. We would prepare by washing down the walls, cleaning, and getting all the unneeded equipment out of the room. They had some instruments and so we did the surgery on the spot at this little hospital.

By contrast, when I was in Taiwan in 1974, I was taken to one of the big national hospitals to work with high-powered reconstructive surgeons. They were keen to do thumb transplants and finger transplants for leprosy, transplanting toes to the hands to replace the digits that patients had worn away. But I considered that quite inappropriate. They had lost fingers because they lacked nerve sensation. They are likely to lose the transferred digits just as they did the original ones. In my experience, when leprosy patients have lost fingers, it is not usually a good idea to try to do such sophisticated replacements.

Nevertheless there are ways we can improve the functions of their hands. Above all, we can teach them to take care of the limb. It is also vital to teach them how to look after themselves **before** any surgery. Without such care, the surgery is really almost a waste of time. It is possible to help improve the function of a hand, say, only to have the patient so misuse it that they destroy it more quickly.

Another interesting place I visited is the Pescadores, a group of 64 small islands in the strait between Taiwan and mainland China. The Portuguese name *Pescadores* means "islands of fishermen". They are very low-lying and windswept, and fishing is indeed the main industry. The capital and largest town is MaKung on Penghu, a fascinating place with its simple village life. There are interesting folk customs and beliefs. The restaurants in Penghu serve whole fish cooked beautifully; you eat the upper side, then you lift the skeleton out and eat the bottom side. You dare not turn your fish over because tradition has it that if you turn a fish over on your plate to get at the other side, then a fishing boat will turn over at sea!

Marjorie Bly met me at the MaKung airport and took me into the city. She was a member of the American Lutheran mission and had been working there for many years. The local health authorities had given her a room in the hospital as her clinic. It meant that, if her patients needed help, she was able to refer them down the passageway to the other specialty clinics in the hospital. In the 60s and 70s she had the assistance of OMF missionary nurse Anne Walker, who spoke a different dialect of Chinese. After working elsewhere with OMF she had been sent to me in Hay Ling Chau to learn something about leprosy before she went to help Marjorie Bly.

Marjorie and Anne used to travel widely by boat and by bus around Penghu, visiting patients in their homes. With them, this was one of the few places where I did home visiting. Marj had the confidence not only of the patients but also of the staff of the local hospital, who thought very highly of her and were only too glad to cooperate. Whenever I went to MaKung, she would have a patient ready with a foot or a hand that needed an operation that I could do with the local surgeons, in the hope of encouraging them to do these things more regularly themselves in future.

One young man was sent to Marjorie as having leprosy. We did not think he had it, so we did a biopsy. He turned out to have a very rare condition for which there was no real treatment. However, while waiting for the biopsy result, Marj had started him on one of the anti-leprosy medications which is also anti-inflammatory, and the lesions subsided well. And so for the next couple of years, every time the lesions flared up, he would come back to Marj for another course of her treatment. Then he would be off on his business again. Other treatments did not eliminate the disease, but with Marj's help he was able to keep it under control and get on with his life.

In the mid-60s I had seen a young woman who had had a foot-drop correction done some years earlier by a visiting surgeon, who had left no instructions for the physiotherapy to be done after the surgery. The surgery itself had been successful but she still walked with the foot-drop, which advertised what her disease was. I spent time with her and then taught Anne what to do to re-educate the transferred tendon to do its job. A good patient and a good teacher; and next time I visited she was very happy to be walking very well, so that others wanted the same procedure. That was the sort of thing one loved to see.

Sadly too, it was another example of how many surgeons are either not trained in post-operative care, or do not leave adequate instructions, and so do not get good results. I am often unable to follow up people I operated on, because by the time I come again, they have gone home. But no news is in most cases good news – if they are not happy they come back!

Marjorie Bly was an amazing woman to work with, very capable, loved by her patients and respected by the local doctors. In later years she had some health troubles, but she stayed at her post in Ma Kung as long as she could. As far as she was concerned, patients were never completely discharged. When they no longer required leprosy medication, she would still get them to come into the clinic every now and again for checks, to make sure their hands and their feet were all right and to see if they needed any other treatment. She was a treasure; it was a treat to work with Marjorie.

Marjorie Bly, Ruth Lin, Rev John Kuo and Gerda Beck were all part of the network of leprosy clinics under the title of the Taiwan Leprosy Relief Association (TLRA). The CEO (as we would call him today) of TLRA in the seventies was David Hsiao, who had an office in Taipei. He was the one who coordinated the various clinics, and helped with hiring new workers and obtaining assistance from American Leprosy Missions, who financially assisted the work in Taiwan. He was involved in the whole upgrading of Taiwan's leprosy programs.

1975 was the beginning of a new era for me, but I was still going to be available to teach the Taiwan workers about leprosy, while fitting Taiwan into a program involving a much wider area of Asia.

The picture for leprosy care in Taiwan has altered dramatically in recent years. The government still tends to understate the number of patients that are affected, but TLRA personnel are convinced that they are seeing fewer patients now and seeing them earlier. Much less deformity is being found in new patients. That is a very big advance.

I continued to visit Taiwan many times, almost every year till 1989. When I made my last visit I was given several very cordial farewell functions and was presented with the Medal of Honour of the National Health Department of Taiwan.

21

Pakistan – the length and the breadth

After leaving Hong Kong in 1974 I flew, via Thailand, into Pakistan. I'd first visited Pakistan in September 1967 (see Chapter 10). It was far too hot for me then. Winter is all right – that is liveable! On this trip I was in Pakistan throughout winter, eight weeks. In the north it was cold.

My tour started in Quetta, Baluchistan, in the west. It is inland and very dry and barren, high on a plateau. The people are known as Baluchis. They do interesting embroidery on their clothing with tiny mirrors inserted into the pattern, held in place by criss-crossed threads.

I stayed near the Mission Hospital in Quetta with the hospital pharmacist and his wife, Mr and Mrs Reg Roberts, a pleasant Australian CMS couple who showed me round the area. There had been snow and it could be so cold at night that vehicles left out all night suffered frozen fuel lines. One man was admitted to the hospital with severe burns because he had tried to light a fire under the engine of his truck to warm it up and get it started!

The hospital had a leprosy clinic staffed by paramedicals from the Marie Adelaide Leprosy Centre (MALC) in Karachi. There were some Afghan patients from over the border, and quite a lot of Baluchis. Some of the severe cases of florid, lepromatous patients that came to Karachi were from this area.

Some years before, in Karachi, I had treated an Afghan patient. She was very badly deformed. Her problems were partly due to leprosy and partly to the fact that she also had a mental deficit and lacked awareness, so she had damaged and destroyed herself unwittingly. Her case illustrated some of the most tragic and intractable elements of leprosy at its worst, in a society where compassion and love were largely lacking – that is, *agape*, love in the Christian sense, which reaches out to the unloved, unlovable and unwanted. At the Marie Adelaide Leprosy Centre we improved her facial appearance somewhat, to make it less repellent. For several years she continued to live at the hospital. There was nowhere else for her to go. She apparently had no relatives; nobody wanted her because of her deformities and disfigurement.

I had a special interest in the way the Baluchis make their bread – their *parn* – in a big circular oven which is heated all round – interested because so many of our patients suffer burns. Because leprosy patients do not feel heat sensation normally, they tend to burn their hands and neglect the wounds. Secondary infection in burns is not uncommon.

Later at Rawalpindi too, I checked on how the women cooked. They would have an open fireplace, usually on the floor with a few bricks or stones beside it to rest implements upon. They had metal 'dixies' – cooking pots – and we had to try to teach patients to use adequate protection, good holders, so that they wouldn't burn themselves. Most of the pots only had metal handles. We taught them to make holders like oven mitts, and squares of padded material. We would also go down to the markets to buy samples of spoons, ladles, lifters and forks with wooden handles so the patients could see suitable, safe implements they could buy.

Back in Karachi I was delighted to meet Dr Thomas Chiang again, working in the Marie Adelaide Leprosy Centre, continuing to learn the craft of caring for leprosy. I soon had him dealing with simple abscesses, infections and foot-drops, and taught him to do some of the face reconstruction surgery.

Then came a lecture tour through the length and breadth of Pakistan.

Despite the prevalence of leprosy, Pakistan, like many other countries, in those days gave little attention to the teaching of leprosy diagnosis or its management in their medical schools and nursing institutions. Most of the medical personnel wouldn't recognise leprosy if they fell over it. Therefore the MALC group wanted me to lecture as widely as possible to students and to associations of graduate doctors. The aim was to foster the teaching of leprosy and also its relevance to problems such as diabetes. They thought people would be more likely to listen to me, as a 'foreign expert', than to one of their own leprosy workers.

We started at Rawalpindi. I discussed how their program, though it had been running quite well, could be improved. Paramedical workers went out from the hospital into the hills and conducted outpatient clinics, but the whole hospital needed to be upgraded.

By 1975 the German sisters were moving from Manghopir to Rawalpindi, as their mission had taken over the management of the Rawalpindi institution and was upgrading it. They employed a capable Pakistani doctor to work there and do the outpatient clinics up in the hills. On this visit I stayed at the Leprosy Hospital in 'Pindi and did some surgery. Sister Adelheide (see chapter 10) had already moved there as physiotherapist and operation room supervisor. They had a well equipped theatre and I operated on many patients in the next few years.

A couple of the local 'Pindi doctors were also interested, and Adelheide arranged for them to come and observe and work with me, assessing and operating. Sometimes I went to operate in their hospitals in the city. The local army dermatologist was also keen to learn, and was most helpful to us. From 1975 I usually lectured in the Army Medical College as well the leprosy hospital. I found that he usually included a question on leprosy in the Dermatologists' Specialist examinations for Pakistan. The work at Rawalpindi over the next few years developed in leaps and bounds.

Among the patients I had seen there in 1969 was a small boy, Sarli, with serious problems. His fingers were shortened and his right ankle had been grossly swollen. Everybody assumed he must have leprosy. He was being treated by one of the Pakistani doctors and I was not confident enough in 1969 to make definite suggestions about dealing with leprosy-like symptoms when the patient did not have leprosy. His right ankle continued swollen and it was assumed that he had osteomyelitis. So in about 1970 he'd had his right leg off – a below the knee amputation. But he continued to develop more problems. By 1975 he had lost all the toes on the other foot, which was partially paralysed. His fingers were getting shorter and shorter. He was literally wearing his fingers away – painlessly. The German sisters brought Sarli to Karachi. I could see that this was not leprosy but I did not know what it was.

At Manghopir Hospital I reconstructed his left foot. I also sent a biopsy of a nerve to a London expert for diagnosis. He confirmed that the boy did not have leprosy at all. He had a "radicular sensory neuropathy", probably congenital. I have since learned that, in many of the third world countries, children can develop these types of problems when their parents are close relatives. There is nothing that can be done about it except to teach the patient and the relatives how to care for their hands and feet. In many respects Sarli was a lucky fellow who had come to probably the only place in Pakistan where he was likely to be properly looked after and taught how to take care of himself.

In his marvellous autobiography *The Gift of Pain,* written with Philip Yancey, Paul Brand says that he once thought of pain as "a blemish in creation, God's one great mistake." As he learnt more and saw the horrendous damage people could do to themselves if, like Sarli, they lacked a normal perception of pain, he realised that, far from being a blemish or a mistake, on the contrary "pain stands out as an extraordinary feat of engineering, valuable beyond measure." (P. 62)

We could not enable Sarli to feel the pain that would protect him, but we did the best we could. When we told his parents that he did not have leprosy, you should have seen the looks on their faces and their absolute change of attitude! They had not wanted him at home when they thought he had leprosy but now that they knew that he did not have it, it was a completely different story. They were then prepared to have him back at home even with all his deformities and multiple problems.

It may have been twenty years later that I met Sarli again in Rawalpindi as an adult. Because of his lack of pain perception he literally had no hands – both were destroyed to above the wrist. Both his legs had been amputated and he lived in a wheelchair – and yet he was a respected member of his community. Sarli ran a taxi service. He was the brains and handled the business, giving all the orders and handling all the planning. This was the boy who had once been condemned as a leper and left in a leprosy hospital, rejected by his family.

The disabled can do so much more than many of us would ever credit. They **are** able. We often say that "where there is a will there is a way" that certainly is true when it comes to some of these people with chronic deformities and disabilities.

At Peshawar in the North-West Frontier I visited and lectured at the Medical College and visited the government leprosy ward in the main teaching hospital. There it was obvious that attitudes and practices needed to be changed. I also visited and did some surgery at the mission hospital where there was another leprosy clinic, and I addressed the local medical practitioners' group.

Then to Abbotabad high in the mountains, with a new and modern medical college. Since then I have lectured there on a number of occasions. I always get a very warm reception from the superintendent, who has had me operating with him on leprosy patients or patients with similar problems. MALC-trained paramedical workers also worked in that area.

On this first occasion I was asked to lecture on leprosy to both the staff and students. I gave a forty-five minute lecture, an overview of leprosy and its care, to an audience of three or four hundred, followed by a question time. After I had been on my feet for about ninety minutes, the principal of the medical college rose to his feet and said, "Dr Warren, I know the answer to this, but would you mind telling my staff and students why Christians do leprosy work?" I saw Sister Adelheide, sitting in the front row, take a gulp.

What a question to throw to me in an auditorium full of mostly Muslim medical personnel! Whereas I usually had to be so careful of religious issues, here I was given an invitation to say that Christians did leprosy work because Jesus Christ had led the way. He had touched and healed people described as having leprosy or other diseases that made them unclean and untouchable in the eyes of their society. He gave us the command not only to care for those who have leprosy but to look after all rejected and needy people. It was a marvellous opportunity and privilege to give a word of witness in a Muslim institution in a country like Pakistan.

There are many Muslims who are prepared to help the poor, the sick and those in need as a means of gaining merit for good works. Well, that occurs in every society. The idea of doing it as a service to Jesus Christ was foreign to them. Jesus (Issa) is regarded as one of their prophets, but not on the same level as Mohammad. On this particular day we were able to show that Jesus led the way. Hopefully some of them will remember why Christians do so much to help leprosy sufferers and the needy in general.

Then I travelled southwards, through the whole length of Pakistan lecturing in virtually all their colleges: the northern ones, Peshawar, Abbotabad, Rawalpindi, in each of which I would lecture on future visits, then Lahore, Lyllapur, Multan and Bahawalaphur.

At Multan, after the lecture, I was asked to see a patient, a man with neuropathy of the hands and feet, for which they could not diagnose the cause. I rapidly did, because he had a perforated nasal septum and no eyebrows, both very common signs of chronic leprosy. He was a typical old lepromatous patient who now had chronic nerve lesions of his arms and his legs. They reckoned they had never had a leprosy patient in their hospital before.

In Bahawalaphur I had to stay in an ordinary hotel – or what we would call a motel. There were many names you could use for this one – the less said the better! Sister Adelheide, who organised my trip, had arranged for some "boys", paramedical workers – to escort me everywhere I went. They were most insistent that I please not leave my room until they came to get me for the next meal or whatever it was, because in Pakistan women never went out unaccompanied. I was rarely welcomed with a handshake because a Muslim man is not meant to touch any woman who is not his wife. Of course women who were strict Muslims were veiled. In respect for their culture, I usually wore a hat or a headscarf when out, and dressed in a Western adaptation of their long tunic tops (kameez) and trousers.

I think that the clothing that I wore was an important reason for the fact that I was so readily accepted. Quite often I'd wear a long skirt when I was lecturing in Karachi because that was acceptable there, but for working with the patients I was happier to wear trousers and tops, especially as in any case I spend half my life down on the floor looking at feet!

My journey followed the Indus River most of its length to the Arabian Sea. We visited a new medical school in Larkana. Then came Hyderabad, Pakistan's second biggest city (there is a Hyderabad in India too), where I had lectured several times before, so I was quite well known and well accepted. Finally I lectured in a number of medical colleges in Karachi itself. For the first time somebody had lectured in every medical college in Pakistan – or all but one; that was omitted because when I got back to Karachi, the Islamic fast month of Ramadan was starting.

Some years later Dr Pfau of MALC advertised for some doctors to join her team. Two young doctors applied for this job. When she questioned them as to what they knew about leprosy she was amazed at how much they seemed to know. "Where did you learn all this?" she asked. They said that when they were medical students a foreign woman came and lectured them. It's reassuring to know that I am not only understood but that I can teach in a manner which can be persuasive as well, so much so that it even convinced those men that it was worthwhile working in leprosy.

I thank God that he has given me the ability to teach. With something like leprosy in Third World countries that is vitally needed. Of course when I am teaching basic care for leprosy, I am also teaching basic care for diabetes and lots of other things which cause similar problems. Being able to help folk with other diseases has meant that many of the younger doctors and surgeons are prepared to have a completely new attitude to leprosy as well. The reconstructive work that I have been doing, remaking hands and feet and faces, and doing it also for patients who have diseases other than leprosy, inclines them to regard leprosy in a much more compassionate and satisfactory light.

After that trip in 1974/75 I spent time in Pakistan approximately every two years for about two to three weeks at a time, working mostly in Karachi, lecturing in various centres and operating. Staff at MALC kept changing, but Dr Thomas Chiang in the 1980s became the CEO of the hospital as well as being the surgeon. He was excellent and not afraid of hard work. So when I was not there he would continue doing the basic routine cases, and he'd save up the more complicated ones for me. The physiotherapy at the centre eventually attained a very good level, as did the shoemaking and the plaster casts. People were sent to India for training in these to benefit the MALC patients.

It was a constant, ongoing program. The paramedical workers

were doing an excellent job in finding new cases, and as a result the number of new patients in Pakistan was falling. The government had organised the program better so that the patients were all registered with their standard identification numbers. It meant they were getting treatment earlier. With fewer deformities developing, not as many new patients needed reconstructive surgery. The whole programme in Pakistan was going extremely well.

However, I was very concerned in the 1990s because I had officially retired from the mission and I wondered about the future of the program. Then, in December 1999, Dr Thomas informed me that a Pakistani hand surgeon, who had recently returned to Karachi from England, had arrived at Marie Adelaide and asked if he could help with the program for the leprosy patients. They suggested that he come to see me. So I met Dr Bhatty, a charming, capable man who had been working in England for some years and who had an English wife. He had a real interest in the patients and their welfare. He was particularly interested in hand surgery for the patients, so I enlisted him to do some.

The next time I visited Karachi, in October 2000, he had arranged to have adequate time off so he could spend a good many days with me doing reconstructive surgery. He was very interested in learning my techniques of doing tendon transfers for the feet, so that he could do them also. We got on extremely well. He could do the face work and was prepared to tackle other plastic surgery procedures when needed.

I hope Dr Bhatty will be able to continue doing the surgery. He is an associate professor in one of the medical colleges, so he has the standing that is needed in Pakistan. He also has the experience and the interests of the patients at heart. He knows the basic principles of what is needed for the leprosy patients, and is better able than I am to assess their needs socially.

Dr Bhatty invited me to go to Pakistan to be a guest speaker at the conference of the Pakistan Hand Surgery Association in November 2001. I had my visa but the September 11 crisis hit and all those plans had to be cancelled. I was advised not go to Pakistan at all at that time. I did get back in February 2004 and we were able to work together again. We also started to train another new MALC staff member to do the routine minor surgery, as Dr Thomas Chiang had left and there was no other senior staff member interested in the surgery.

I am hopeful that Dr Bhatty will be able to carry on doing what is necessary, but I am pretty sure that he would like me to go back so that we could have that level of discussion and sharing which is so important when one is dealing with problems as complicated as the reconstruction of hands. He is quite prepared to do some surgery for feet as well and for this I am grateful.

I was able to return in 2005 when I was one of the invited guests at the Pakistan Hand and Plastic Surgeons' Conference. There they acknowledged how much I had done since 1967 in the reconstructive surgery for leprosy patients. I left Pakistan at the end of February 2005 and flew home via Thailand, arriving in time to receive, on 10th March, an email saying, in effect, "Your name has been proposed for the national awards in Islamabad for 23rd March. Can you come back?" Well, there was no time for me to secure a visa and a ticket and get to Islamabad by the 23rd. So they said I could receive it in Canberra. That is another story.

22

Burma – Smugglers' Tales

In February 1975, from Karachi, I flew into Burma for the first time.

Burma had been a closed country for years, but in the early 1970s the doors began to creak open. Originally, people were able to get visas for one or two nights only. Missionaries and linguists involved in Bible translation would do as much as they could outside of Burma. When necessary they would dash into Rangoon for an overnight stay at a hotel, meet up with their language informants and literally work all night. Then they'd leave Burma and continue their work outside its borders.

I was able to obtain a tourist visa for two weeks, and took a 40-minute flight south to Moulmein, where The Leprosy Mission had a hospital. If you do not fly it is a good 12-hour train trip, plus another hour to reach a river, cross by ferry and then go by car to the city.

Moulmein is where the American Adoniram Judson (1788-1850) did a lot of his Bible translation. He was one of the early missionaries into Burma, a gifted linguist who soon became fluent in Burmese and translated much of the Bible into the Burmese tongue, translations that are still being used today. He is a well known figure in Burmese history, not only in the history of the Christian Church there.

The mission hospital at Moulmein was originally built in about 1890. It has an attractive chapel with stained glass windows where morning prayers, attended by staff and patients, are held daily. Most of the buildings are simple and basic, but adequate. Being a tropical country Burma has tropical downpours but rarely any cold weather. The Burmese are used to sleeping on the floor on a bed-mat and do not require mattresses. In the hospital we had bedsteads with wooden boards instead of mattresses. The patients put their bed-mats on those boards. This they found perfectly comfortable, so who were we to object?

What it did mean was that we did not have to provide sheets. In Burma in the 1970s, that was a big plus because there were severe restrictions on the availability of any woven material. The government rationed fabrics so that each Burmese citizen was allowed to purchase two, and only two, longees each year, and two blouses. A longee is the long skirt that men and women wear, all day every day. It goes from the waist to the ankle, similar to the Thai garment the *pa.*

If they needed more longees, they were available – at a price – on the black market. Moumein was close to the Thai/Burmese border. The smugglers' trails led into Moulmein, and at the city's edge was a big market where people could buy these goods at a relatively cheap price. Then to get them from Moulmein north to Rangoon was another problem. The train did not actually come to Moulmein. One had to cross the river by ferry, and then climb a steep hill to the station where one could get a train for the 12 hour trip to Rangoon (Yangon as they call it today).

On several of my trips to Moulmein in the 1980s, I had to take a Burmese tourist guide with me. Security was getting tighter, and also the government had discovered that this was a way of making money. A couple of times I had, as a guide, a young woman who was meant to keep me in her sight at all times. But she left me to my own devices and scarcely bothered at all with surveillance. On another trip, from Moulmein to Rangoon, I had a man as a tourist guide. No, he did not insist on sharing my room – but we had to stay in the same hotel. We had to leave at 5 am to get the boat and catch the 6 am train.

At the railway station there was panic in the air. The customs officials were having a field day. They were checking everybody's possessions to see who was carrying illicit goods bought in the black markets near Moulmein. I realised that the people in the carriage had been secreting their goods everywhere. The officials were collecting all the obvious black market stuff on the railway platforms in piles of confiscated goods. One woman had lost bolts and bolts of material, and, all the way to Rangoon, she bewailed her loss.

We discovered that we ourselves were sitting on top of somebody's purchases, stowed under our seats. When the guard came through, my tour guide carefully said to him about me, "Oh, no, she is a tourist. No, she hasn't got anything. She hasn't been shopping, she has been at the hospital." And so the guard did not worry about what I was sitting on – someone else's black market goods. Even the tourist guide was unwittingly sitting on some too. Along the line passengers would throw things out to people waiting at the crossings or sidings, to avoid being caught with these goods. Train travel through Burma was interesting to say the least!

But to get back to Moulmein. Though the old hospital had been built years before, it was in reasonably good repair. It was simple and clean. It was efficiently run with basic requirements, but the doctor in charge, Dr John Edwards, desperately lacked adequate medications and supplies to do his job.

John was born in Rangoon where his father, in the 1920s, had been the Superintendent of Police. John went through medical school in Burma, and was working in a clinic up in the border areas when the Japanese moved in and occupied the country in 1942. He had had an accident as a child and one leg had been amputated above the knee. When the Japanese came into that hospital all the doctors but John had fled, so they asked him, "Why did not you run away too?" He pulled up his trouser leg and said, "How do you think I can run with this thing!" He was a POW for the rest of the war and had to help care for the Japanese soldiers and any of the prisoners that they had taken.

John Edwards had been working with the mission for many years doing what he could for leprosy patients at Moulmein. He was officially a Burmese citizen, but had a British passport too. Originally he had had reasonable supplies and had attempted some research into drug and general treatment of leprosy. However, by the time I saw him he was very short of everything, and it was very difficult for him to get hold of suitable medications for his patients, or even to get the proper anti-leprosy drugs. But he carried on loyally as best he could.

He greeted me very warmly. I was the first foreigner to visit his hospital for many years. At last somebody had come who could share with him the up-to-date treatments of leprosy and modern ways of doing things. So we talked a great deal, saw patients and I did a bit of surgery. I also went down to the government hospital at Moulmein and gave a lecture there on leprosy to the other doctors and the nurses in the town.

John had a very charming and much younger Chinese wife, Ma Yu, and we benefited from the fact that her brother was a very good Chinese cook. I lived in the house with John, his wife and their two delightful little children. Every afternoon, when we arrived home from the hospital, which was just across the road from their home, Ma Yu would have a fresh coconut for me. She'd found out that I liked drinking sparkling fresh green coconut milk and would send one of the boys up a tree.

There were leprosy patients at all stages of the disease. One girl had very bad eye problems and John was unable to get the right treatment for her. I was able to get the German leprosy group to send in some medication for her, and later was able to send medication from Thailand so John could continue treating her. Aspirin is, of course, very commonly available to us. It's cheap and widely used and we do not even think of its importance. But in Burma at that time aspirin was expensive black market contraband.

People just could not afford to buy tablets for toothache, pain or fever.

John's wife, Ma Yu, used to give out medication and do the dispensing; they did not have a fully qualified pharmacist. A lot of the medicines that they wanted, they could not get. For drugs that were to be taken once daily, especially those that were expensive such as steroids, we made sure that Ma Yu saw the tablet actually swallowed, so we knew that the patient could not go and sell it.

Many leprosy patients had bad skin conditions. No cortisone cream was available. But zinc oxide powder was obtainable as was sump oil from motor vehicle engines. So we concocted a horrid looking brew of white zinc powder mixed into blackish brown oily stuff which could be rubbed on skin lesions. Yes, it did work!

Ma Yu ran a "feeding station". The Christian Blind Mission provided the funds and Ma Yu organised a band of volunteer helpers. John built a big shed as a dining room, and every morning they served a decent breakfast to the children of leprosy patients and others in need – better than giving the parents the money as it could go on drink or drugs.

In 1977 I traveled north to Mandalay, and at the leprosy hospital there met Ruth and Ken Thein. Ken was a Burmese physiotherapist who had been sent to India in 1960 to learn the physiotherapy of leprosy. His teacher in India was an Englishwoman, Ruth Thomas, and thereby hangs a tale – they married and Ruth returned with Ken to Burma. She became a Burmese citizen and spent the rest of her life there working with him in the leprosy programs.

At Mandalay, an excellent leprosy physiotherapy programme was under way. There was an orthopaedic surgeon who was doing some of the surgery. He greatly appreciated the opportunity of being able to talk with me, to discuss problems and learn techniques. He also showed me around the general hospital, and my heart went out to them in pity, because of the limited facilities. People in Australia comment on how I 'make do'. But in Burma, they were forced to 'make do' far more.

An orthopaedic surgeon was doing hip replacements by having the head of a femur – the long bone of the leg – carved out of ivory, so he could insert it in patients who had suffered that fracture when a metal implant was not available. Seeing the waste of appliances and equipment that occurs in Australia, and realising what these people are making do with, how much they improvise, really makes one sad. There is so much sheer waste in developed countries and we fail to give more to these people who are in such need.

In Mandalay there were lots of little things I could help with. I went to Mandalay several times over the next four or five years. Each time, my suitcase would be loaded with surgical sutures. The Burmese government stated that it provided the surgical sutures that the surgeons required in Government hospitals, but only after a lot of red tape. When a surgeon needed a packet of sutures, he had to be able to hand in an equivalent number of needles to show he had used the last lot. So I could make a surgeon extremely happy when I arrived with extra packets of sutures or needles. This surgeon, a compassionate and dedicated man, was very willing to try to help the patients with deformities. As a result there were numerous patients around Mandalay whose successful hand and foot operations enabled them to work and support themselves and their families.

I was also able to arrange for the German Leprosy Association to send in to Ken Thien the drug Lamprene which was still very expensive and unavailable in Burma, where there were many patients who badly needed it. From Thailand I managed to send in packets of leprosy drugs, Lamprene, dapsone, and later, rifampicin, so that the patients could get the best possible medication.

Not far from the leprosy hospital in Moulmein was a "leprosy village" where many affected people lived. There were dozens of children, and John and Ma Yu Edwards regularly checked them for evidence of the disease.

The children of Burma usually have olive skin, so leprosy appears as light patches on their skin. These are a warning. If the patches completely disappear over the next six months it shows the child's own immune system has acted and clinical disease is unlikely to develop. However, in a small proportion of children the patches do not go away. Some will end up getting more and more patches. They do not hurt. The child does not feel sick, but he does have leprosy. In this village I took many photographs, and, in my sets of teaching slides many of the early lesions that I show have come from that particular village: patches of all sizes and shapes and stages of healing.

I was able speak to the doctors and nurses at the Rangoon general hospital and share with them some of what I knew of leprosy. I also did some lecturing for the leprosy team in Rangoon on some trips and saw some of the surgery done there. Burma was actually ahead of some of the other Asian countries in organizing the district nurses to run the health clinics in the villages and districts. These nurses had received some instruction as to how to look after leprosy.

My ability to do reconstructive surgery was very much appreciated. On that first trip we operated on one or two patients at the Moulmein leprosy hospital. On another trip I worked at the government general hospital, using their equipment to do reconstructive work on the hand of one of the Buddhist monks. When monks greet one another they put their palms together with their fingers straight. So a leprosy-deformed hand is a real and obvious disability. In Thailand I'd learnt that if a person has leprosy he will not be accepted as a novice in a monastery. However, if he develops leprosy after he is already a monk, then he is not turned out. The Thai believe that if you have leprosy it is because you had done something wrong in a previous existence; you could be regarded as a person of low morality, best avoided.

Sometimes the government kept their eye on me. Once we were tailed at a distance wherever we went. Flying out of Burma was also quite a game because you had to go through very close security checks. In particular you were not allowed to take out Burmese money. Kyats had to remain in Burma. On entering Burma one had to register one's camera and check it again when leaving. On my second trip I had a new camera for Dr John Edwards. But we took care. We made sure that it was the same type, same brand as his old one. I listed the brand on my form, and when I went out I had a broken camera of the same brand, so all was well!

As I've said, John was sadly in need of medical supplies. We found a couple of interesting ways of helping. First of all it was not illegal to take in bandages, nor was it illegal to send things in by post as long as the parcel did not weigh more than one kilogram. Then it was delivered to the hospital with no questions asked. If it was more than a kilogram, it went into customs and was assessed and they would charge duty on it. So in Thailand I would collect aspirin, leprosy drugs, eye medications, ointments, antibiotics, etc., remove all the packaging and do them up in plastic bags and post in a few packets weighing less than a kilogram several times a week. The Australian Red Cross kept us supplied with many medicines for Burma from their 'donated supplies division' that has now closed. At least we were able to maintain a supply of the essentials.

A senior customs officer at the Rangoon airport was found to be sympathetic to the leprosy patients' needs. Thereafter we made sure that I always came in on a flight when he was on duty. I made quite sure he knew I was coming on that flight, so that when I came up to the customs counter he would tell one of the officials that he could trust to open my bags. Invariably, when we opened the cases, rolls of bandages would fall in all directions from at least one of the bags, for the leprosy patients. So, duty-bound, that official would go back and report that I was bringing in gifts of bandages and medicines for the leprosy patients, and he would say 'That's fine. That's all right. She can take those.' Every time I went to Burma I think I had between 80 and 100 kilos of medical supplies of all sorts. Thai Airlines, with whom I regularly flew, usually granted me 100 kg excess baggage free because it was donated by the Red Cross! Only once in the ten years when I went in and out of Burma every year did we have to pay duty: it was quite a considerable amount, and took months for them to clear.

So God looks after his own. God gets his supplies through. He has his own people in the right place at the right time so that his work can be carried out.

Many of the bandages I used to carry were knitted from a good cotton yarn. They wash well, they wear well, they are strong and are very easy for the patient to apply. When the bandages arrive at a hospital in Burma, they are eagerly looked over, because if a staff member or a patient can find three or four bandages of the same sort of cotton material, they will undo them, wash them, and then knit them up into a sleeveless sweater, to supplement their meagre clothing ration.

I mentioned earlier that Burmese beds do not have sheets. Nevertheless, a group of ladies in Romania, who were TLM supporters, for years, bought nicely coloured drip-dry bed sheets which, when wrapped, weighed less than one kilogram. Every week they would wrap up one bed sheet and post it to the Leprosy Hospital. Now a bed sheet is a nice piece of material, wide and long enough to make a perfect longee. So when enough of these sheets had arrived they would supply them to a group of nurses or staff. The men all had blue longees and the women had pink or green ones, all made from these bed sheets. So the ladies in Romania provided the staff with their uniforms!

I found the Burmese a lovely people to work with. I enjoyed my days in Burma. In keeping with the social mores I obliged by wearing a longee, or the Thai equivalent, when I was there. I thoroughly enjoyed wandering around Rangoon, which was a very cosmopolitan city. I felt quite safe. I used my bits of Chinese at the markets, and I also found there were lots of second hand bookshops where I could buy cheap but interesting reading matter.

As I went in and out of Burma for ten years I found that it became more and more difficult to travel freely. Eventually it became just too difficult for me to continue to visit regularly, so I had to give up my work in Burma. No leprosy consultant has been able to take my place. But our workers continue as best they can.

23

Changing Routines: Hay Ling Chau Closes

Our major outreach from Hong Kong in the 1960s and early 70s was to Malaysia and Singapore. By the mid-seventies there was much less need for me to go there as they now had their own physiotherapists and had developed their own surgery and rehabilitation programs.

In Singapore, so much had been accomplished in ten years that in leprosy the surgeons were virtually done out of a job. Up to ten of the government surgeons had worked with me, one or two at a time, and they continued operating without me between visits. They realised that the reconstructive surgery experience they were gaining could be of inestimable value in their general work, as it is applicable to accidents, polio and other medical problems. The turnover of government surgeons was high. But once they had private practices they could not work in the government leprosy hospital.

Singapore had little in the way of government social assistance or pensions, so patients who had reconstructive surgery lacked financial support to cover their convalescence and rehabilitation. Hence many decided against having the surgery if they could manage without it. After the mid-1970s, I still went there on occasion to see patients, to advise and to give lectures.

In Malaysia it was somewhat different. The Superintendent of Sungei Buloh Leprosy Hospital, Dr Bjowani, with whom I had worked for over ten years, had retired and returned to India, and the doctor who took over from him did not really know me. I met the new superintendent in the early 80s at a leprosy conference in Chiang Mai. He was obviously very interested to learn that in the past I had been in and out of Sungei Buloh, helping with the surgery for their patients. He said that he wanted me to go back there. Knowing the Asian mind, I said, "When you get back to Malaysia, if you want me to come, please write me a letter of invitation." The last thing I wanted to do was to foist myself upon people, operating on their patients and using their equipment, if they did not want me there. If they wanted to learn – fine – I would go and teach. If not, it would be a waste of my time and theirs. That invitation to return to Sungei Buloh never came. I do not think I went back there after 1976.

Dr Michael Waters, who had been doing medical work at Sungei Buloh for many years, went back to London to work at the Hospital for Tropical Diseases. So he was not there to invite me to come back into his unit either. I had enjoyed the sessions with Michael and learnt a lot of the medical side of leprosy from him. I worked again with him in England in the years 1978 to 1994. Michael has continued to be my leprosy medical mentor, and, even today, I will phone him up in UK to discuss the best way to manage some unusual medical situation in one of my leprosy patients.

In 1975, the last of the Hay Ling Chau patients were moved away from the island to live in the resettlement blocks in Hong Kong. The hospital, which we had been running for over twenty years, was being taken over by the government for use in treating drug addicts. They certainly wouldn't be doing surgery there. We knew full well that there were many other leprosy hospitals that could use the equipment, the instruments and everything else from our hospital.

In the 1970s, I had been the adviser to the British Army on the management of Ghurkhas who had leprosy. The Ghurkhas, from Nepal, formed a well-known British regiment and were posted in Hong Kong. Some of them were discovered to have leprosy and required treatment. However, because few of the British army doctors had ever seen leprosy, they made some enquiries of Dr Waters in Malaysia and he advised them to have me as consultant.

So I made a number of trips to the British Army Hospital in Kowloon. Once they even gave me a helicopter air-lift with a Chinese leprosy patient who needed urgent care. As we were closing down, they were most cooperative and wanted to know what they could do to help. They asked where all the equipment was to go.

Well, there was a TLM hospital in Nepal which could well use a lot of the equipment. Where could be more appropriate than Nepal, with the Ghurkha connection? The British Army volunteered to fly operating tables, lights, instruments, drapes, sheets – you name it – in their Hercules transport planes into Kathmandu, then transport it up to the leprosy hospital at Anandaban. This was an absolute gift because we did not have to pay any transport or shipping costs or even packing costs, and there were no problems with the immigration and customs. We thanked God, while the army did it all for us!

But I had the job of sorting and preliminary packing. So early in 1975, after my trip to Pakistan and Burma, I went back to Hong Kong. I attended a couple of leprosy clinics and went over to the island on several occasions, packing up the equipment and arranging what should go to Nepal. I also claimed some surgical items which I knew I could carry and use myself, and sent some other equipment to wherever we thought it would be most useful.

An interesting development concerned my old school friend Kathleen Collett, who had worked in Malaysia with CMS. The Malaysian government introduced a time limit for expatriates to work in Malaysia because of their policy of "Malayanisation" of all positions following independence. Kathleen had gone to Malaya in 1955 and her time was up in 1968. An English nurse retired and Kathleen was then able to transfer to Hay Ling Chau to work with us – an ideal appointment as she already spoke Cantonese. I valued her support and friendship in the midst of all the problems, and the opportunity to discuss with her the many decisions that I needed to make in those final years up to closure. Then she was out of a job, but not for long. She was offered a position in the big Christian Nethersole Hospital in Hong Kong, as Nurse Counsellor and mentor of the trainee nurses.

So when I went back to Hong Kong in 1975, Kathleen was working at Nethersole and Alan and Rena Waudby were also still there. Alan, as our administrative superintendent, needed to remain until all the equipment was ready to despatch; he had to deal with a lot of red tape. It was rather hard going back to the island when there were no patients, when the hospital had been stripped of so many familiar things. Yet it would still be used as a hospital. Though many changes were in progress on the island, the chapel would remain and still be used, and our Chinese pastor, Mr Leung Sing Sang, would continue to go out on Saturday mornings to conduct services for any of the residents who wished to attend.

We were interested to go back for other reasons. We had made many good friends in Hong Kong and one of them was Gloria Baretto. She worked for Mr Kadoorie, who ran a big agricultural program in the New Territories, on the Kowloon peninsula. There he was trying to collect all the different varieties of plants indigenous to Hong Kong. One of these was a remarkable orchid, *Eulophia Flava*, which grew on the island. It was leafless in winter and then up would come a thick green leaf, then one flower stem per bulb, which grew about a metre high with brilliant yellow flowers. Among the trees we found some bulbs, and also another tiny pink orchid. We were delighted to find these plants to give to Gloria so they would be preserved for posterity, growing in the plant repository.

Despite these minor botanical enterprises our stay in Hong Kong in 1975 was brief. It was really only a transit spot to pack up the last of my goods as I set off on my way back to Taiwan for the first of my trips in the new way of working. After Taiwan I made a short stop at Manorom to collect supplies for a visit I was making to Burma.

In August 1975 I went back to India, on one of the early visits in a whole series of visits to Indian centres over the next five to ten years. I had been asked to go to Purulia to assist with the surgical program. Purulia is a leprosy hospital with a very long history. It is well over 100 years old and is a well established centre. Some of the old brick buildings have since been replaced with new ones provided by gifts from Rotary International and various other charity organizations. It is the centre for a large outreach work, dealing with literally thousands of leprosy patients in the surrounding districts. The staff travel out every day in four-wheel drive vehicles to conduct clinics under trees, in houses, at government hospitals – wherever leprosy patients can be diagnosed and treated.

Many of the paramedical workers who are attached to Purulia live at their clinics in the villages so that they can supervise the treatment and ensure that the patients take their medicines; one of the biggest problems we have to face is non-compliance of patients taking their medicine. At Purulia there are dozens of patients who expect to live there for years. Many have their own houses and their children have gone to school there. A nearby large village consists almost entirely of ex-leprosy patients.

With a hospital of that size, there is every variety of patient needing help. There are also a number of non-leprosy patients. We were able to help children with club feet and similar problems by means of surgery. The hospital was staffed by Indians, and, at the time I first went there, Dr Kiran Das was in charge of the surgical program. Kiran is the daughter of Victor Das, who had been TLM director for India. Kiran had gone through medicine with a TLM scholarship so that she could come back and work in our leprosy programs.

She had then married, and her husband was working in a bank in Purulia. So it was ideal for Kiran to be on our hospital staff. She had been doing some of the routine surgery, but there was much more that could be done and many patients at Purulia had problem feet.

In the 1960s, the commonly accepted method of looking after grossly deformed feet was to have the shoemakers custom-make orthopaedic boots. Unfortunately these boots were difficult to make and therefore expensive. They also had to be replaced at regular intervals. A really active person would need more than one pair of boots every year. Another important thing was that to prevent ulceration, the patient must never take a single step without his boots – and should put them on even at night when getting up to go to the toilet – certainly an inconvenience! So of course many patients did not bother, and their deformed feet ended up with ulcerations on the sites which the shoes were made to protect.

The work we did in Hong Kong altered the whole concept of this, because what we showed in Hong Kong and what was included in my Master of Surgery thesis, (1972), was that this type of deformity can be corrected by surgery. Older text books, especially pre-1950, will say that it cannot be corrected and this is the prognosis that many orthopaedic surgeons still give. If they see a foot with this gross bone abnormality which is so typical, not only of leprosy feet but of diabetic feet and others, they may tell the patient they have an incurable Charcot foot. Whereas we know that properly treated, these bones *will* heal and the patient shouldn't need to be condemned to a deformed foot and an orthopaedic boot for the rest of his or her life.

In Purulia in 1976 this surgical cure had not yet been applied and there were many patients with deformed feet. Some had orthopaedic shoes and others were waiting for special shoes to be made. My job at Purulia in those days was to advise, to see what could be done and to teach Kiran and the other members of the staff the surgical techniques which were applicable to these patients under their care.

An English physiotherapist, Margaret, was very skilled, and was kept very busy teaching national technicians the appropriate physiotherapy. Although there was a Physiotherapy School in India, there were not as yet many graduates, and leprosy certainly wouldn't be one of their chosen specialties, so very few fully qualified physiotherapists did leprosy work in India. Margaret also taught the technicians how to make cheap plaster of paris bandages, because in those days in India we could not afford to buy ready-made, imported expensive plaster bandages. We could buy the powder relatively cheaply, so one of the jobs to be done at the hospital was to make plaster of paris bandages. One needed to put on more layers, making the plaster heavier and it did not last as long, especially in humid conditions. But it was effective.

Most of the Indian surgeons would have trained at Lahore or Karigiri with input from Paul Brand and Ernest Fritschi, two of the TLM senior surgeons. Paul had written about the tarsal bone lesions – the bone disintegration lesions – that are the common problem in both leprosy and diabetes. Both Paul and Ernest wrote about using special callipers, braces and long splints which take the weight from the knee instead of the foot. But they also implied that, once there is a severe deformity, there is not much that can be done about it.

One year a young boy was sent down to us in Purulia from Bhutan. He had many deformities – hands and feet and face. We were working on these, and, on one of my trips, I reconstructed a foot, to try and give it a better shape. I left strict instructions when I left, that that foot was to be kept in a plaster cast till I came back. It was not Dr Kiran Das who was in charge at that stage. Another surgeon, who had not worked with me, did not comply, the boy was taken out of my plaster very early and the foot just broke again, which was what I had feared would happen if that was done.

I could see that it was no use trying to do that type of surgery with that particular doctor in charge. The boy was then sent down to Dr Fritschi in Karigiri – and sent back with a pair of boots. I never will understand why the foot was not reconstructed to give that boy the most useful foot possible for the rest of his life. Just think of the problems of sending him back to Bhutan relying on specially made orthopaedic boots! It was just not practical. Who was going to make the next pair? A growing boy was going to need boots probably every six months!

This was the sort of problem that we were constantly up against with leprosy patients. They needed special footwear made regularly, or else they needed their feet reconstructed. A few of the bad ones needed both. The feet of the majority of these patients could be reconstructed so that they could wear the type of shoes that were available freely on the open market and did not require to be constantly provided by our special shoemakers.

Over the next ten years, I taught quite a number of people these reconstruction techniques. This trip was the beginning of an ongoing relationship with a number of different centres in India where I was able to work with many different Indian surgeons, hopefully helping them to learn more and to appreciate more of what could be done to save the feet of leprosy patients.

I made short trips to a number of TLM hospitals and centres to try and help improve standards. Most were staffed by Indians, not expatriates. But early on I visited Champa and worked with Dr Ian Cochrane and his wife Marion, from the UK. That was probably the first time I worked with Ian. Later he went to Purulia Hospital and did the surgery there and later still I worked with him in Bangladesh.

24

New Base – Thailand

After 1975 the OMF Manorom Christian Hospital in central Thailand was the base from which I operated as a roving ambassador caring for leprosy patients. But I worked in other places in Thailand too.

When at Manorom I occupied a large room with its own en suite, right in the hub of the hospital. Most of my time was spent looking after the leprosy patients. There was a large clinic every Thursday with maybe over 100 patients. A lot of them had foot problems that needed to be treated. The patients were taught self-care, and the older patients would teach the new ones.

It was interesting to look back to 1963 when I had stayed there for three months. Then there were lots more problem feet, but many patients had now learnt to look after themselves. Much of that advance was due to one of the patients that I had seen on the first trip. (See chapter 10 page 83)

There was also Mr Yen, originally a patient for foot-drop correction. While there, waiting to have his cast off, he too started helping other patients. Before long he had quite a clientele. He taught ulcer care, self-care and exercises. He had little education but he was a lovely fellow, who had come to know Christ and was transformed because of what the Christian nurses and Manorom Hospital had done for him. He was so useful and reliable that we kept him on for years as a patient/staff member. We could rely on him for the routine physiotherapy teaching. If a patient needed a plaster cast, Yen would get the plaster ready for us to put on and then clean up the mess after us. A wonderful ministry – nothing seemed too much bother for him.

The OMF also had a hospital at Saiburi in the far south of the peninsula towards Malaysia, an area with a mainly Muslim population. That program started originally as clinics, but then a weatherboard hospital was built. The nearby government hospital did not really want the problems of leprosy patients, so the Saiburi Christian Hospital provided a centre for treating leprosy and some of the community's general medical needs.

After 1975 I went to Saiburi every few months for a week or two, to attend their medical clinics and to do surgery. Dr David Simpkin from Australia was there as the surgeon for part of that time. Together we would see the patients and do some surgery, with his wife Marjorie doing the physiotherapy. David did general surgery too, including repairing children's hare lips and cleft palates.

There we encountered some very interesting patients. Diagnosis was sometimes a problem because people came in with very mixed symptoms only partly typical of leprosy. A young boy had had surgery in one of the government hospitals, for a cyst in his knee which had destroyed the nerve which activated the muscles that lift the foot. So he had a foot-drop just like leprosy. We operated on him and removed more of the cyst, and corrected his foot-drop. He was thrilled to regain a reasonably normal gait. There were many situations like this – patients with leprosy-like problems which we could deal with using leprosy techniques.

Pattani was a bigger centre nearby with a clinic where many of the patients came for diagnosis, and for treatment including their anti-leprosy medication. There I stayed with Brenda Holton, an English OMF nurse who was expert in leprosy and had been treating it for years. With OMF input and encouragement, that clinic, which Brenda ran with another nurse, became the headquarters of the local Christian church. Some leprosy patients became leaders in the church and helped with the translation of the Bible and Christian books into the local variant of the Malay language.

There were two Thai paramedical workers; the younger man was doing his best to learn English, while the other was a Malay-speaking Muslim. This gave him entrance into their communities, enabling us to contact Muslim patients and win their confidence. The men rode motor bikes in and out of the villages, looking for patients who had not turned up for treatment, doing dressings and routine treatments. It was a good set-up, and many of those patients were able to thank God for the fact that the Christian church had set up a hospital which would give to them the care they needed.

Now that I was regularly in Thailand, the Government Leprosy Hospital at Phrapradaeng in Bangkok wanted me to visit more often. It was a very big institution – it had been there for many years and as usual in the early days the leprosy patients admitted expected never to go home. Then we started doing reconstructive surgery, particularly for foot-drop. Surgery could thus eliminate the obvious signs of the disease and the reason for their staying in the hospital long-term was gone.

Some patients wanted to be discharged, but there was another group who did not want that at all. They were living in quite reasonable accommodation. Food, clothing and a small amount of pocket money were provided. By the standards of poorer people in Thailand they were secure and quite well off. Why leave when they did not have to? Therefore many of these patients when offered surgery refused it. They could manage as they were, thank you!

Nevertheless, a lot of operations were done. In my earlier days there, Dr Ake Chardtong was in charge of the surgery. Dr Ake had been a fellow student with me at Karigiri in India in 1963, together with two other Thai doctors, Dr Teira and Dr Somphorn.

Thailand has an excellent Old Boys' Club; if you were a student with somebody, there is an unwritten code that you get preferred treatment in your dealings with them. So having been at Karigiri with these three doctors, I found that when I went to Thailand to work, they were all very helpful. Dr Ake was very pleased for me to come and help with the surgery. The others also had senior positions and I was frequently invited to official meetings and government ceremonies.

In 1975, the Government was tightening up on various requirements, and one of the new restrictions was that doctors could not be registered to work in Thailand unless they sat for their exams in Thai. For me, the Leprosy Division of Thailand organised a special modified registration which allowed me to do leprosy work anywhere in Thailand, without my having to sit for that exam. Just as well! One of the senior OMF missionaries, who had worked for many years in China, was probably well into his 70s when he had to do this exam. The young Thai doctor examining him started off with a ridiculously simple question, and when the doctor started to answer, the examiner said, "Don't worry about that, you know far more about it than I do. It's OK, we will pass you!"

At Phrapradaeng Dr Ake would call in patients with all sorts of problems, paralysis and deformities. We would discuss what could be done, and some of them he would put on his own list and say "Right, I will do that!" About others he would say to me, "Oh, I do not know how to do that; will you come and teach my trainees?" A statement like that from any Asian specialist was very unusual. Dr Ake's realistic humility was refreshing.

I spent many days there, operating on his patients. He also invited me to lecture the staff on leprosy. Once I remonstrated with him and said, "You're quite capable of teaching that!" "Oh well" he said, "I might be, but the staff will listen to you much more than they will listen to me!" Dr Ake also took me to a fairly new leprosy hospital at Khon Kaen in the north-east. We did some of the first reconstructive surgery there.

One year, Dr Ake invited me to deliver a series of teaching programs, daily from December 23 to 27. December 23 was a Monday. I was living with a houseful of Christian nurses and we all had different rosters. We had agreed that we would have our Christmas dinner on Saturday night 28th because of various duties over the Christmas period. We could then relax and enjoy a celebration dinner together. Accordingly I did not say anything to him about Christmas and agreed to do the series. On Monday and Tuesday we had full mornings of lectures and afternoons of demonstrations. Wednesday was Christmas Day. We assembled, and Dr Ake, looking embarrassed, apologised most profusely that he had forgotten the date was 25th December, our special feast day. And he presented me with a beautiful piece of patterned green Thai silk.

I took the opportunity of explaining that yes, this was a special day but it was not a day that **had** to be celebrated on 25th December – that we had planned to have our special dinner and feast on the Saturday. We were still able to celebrate that Jesus Christ had come to earth for humanity's sake. Whether we celebrated his birth on the 25th December or any other stated day, the main thing was that we wanted to recognise the one who was born to be the Saviour of the world. So I thanked him for the gift and we got on with the lecture.

This showed the type of man that Dr Ake was. One lovely trait of his, which one does not always find in Asians, was realising that there were lots of things which other people could probably do better than he could. The rarity of this perception is one of the things that I have had to live with over the years. Particularly with Asians, one must be wary of status and sensitivities, especially with regard to what one has been taught. One must try to avoid criticizing people in front of others and making them 'lose face' (that is the term that they use). Their embarrassment may make them feel that they would have to avoid you or that situation in the future. The other thing is that it is culturally extremely difficult to say "No." If they do want to do something, they can say "Yes" and mean it. But if they do not want to do it, they often find it very difficult to refuse. If you ask an Asian to do something, he (or she) will rarely say that he cannot do it. He may attempt it and make a mess of it but then you cannot directly criticise him. So you need to be very careful in how you do things, and what you encourage them to do. For instance, it is very difficult and embarrassing to have to ask a surgical trainee to undo wrongly placed stitches!

Long before I went to Phrapradaeng, I had developed a method of avoiding problems like this with my Asian colleagues. I was often asked to demonstrate a certain operation with lots of people looking on. I would be trying to teach one of their surgeons how to do a procedure like a foot-drop correction. I cannot embarrass him by correcting him in front of the others if he does not do it right. So I developed a patter, a spiel. I would make it clear first that the Asian doctor was actually doing the operation, but that I would be there to help him. I would give a detailed running description of the whole procedure as it was done so that before a move was actually made, I was informing everyone what we were going to do next and the pros and cons of why one did it this way rather than that way. I was able to help them and to teach without embarrassing them. In fact I found it rather fun to teach in this way.

I know that some of the Asians I taught went on to do these procedures for others – not only for leprosy patients, because the types of tendon transfers that I do have a far wider use than just for leprosy.

When Dr Ake had to retire a much younger man was appointed. He felt that he knew it all and did not really appreciate what I was doing. So once he took over I did not do nearly as much surgery, though I still did some of the general leprosy work.

I made many good friends. One of the staff that I still contact regularly is Mr Somkiet, a physiotherapist who is most meticulous in how he looks after his patients. He is so appreciative of what we can do to help and it is he who quite often encourages me to go back there to work. He also supervises the shoemakers and the orthotic

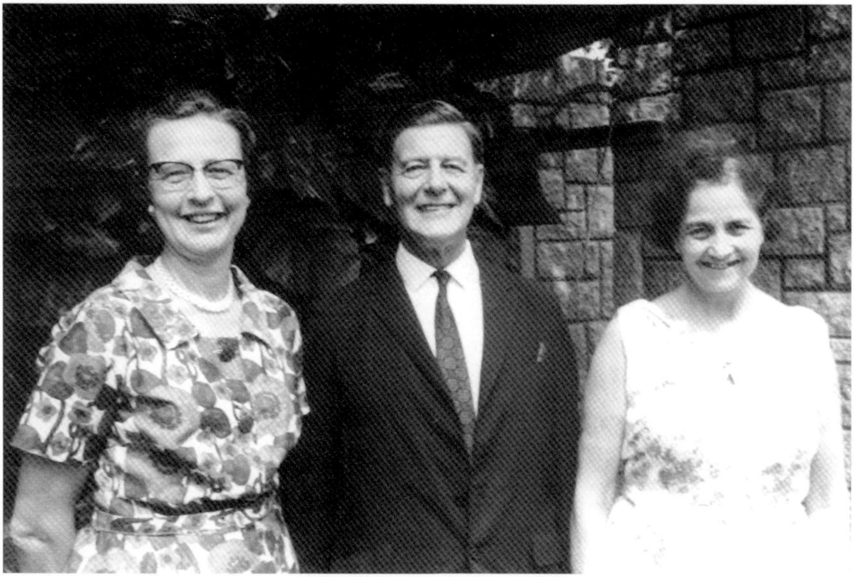

Dr Grace with Dr Stanley & Mrs Mali Browne - 1972

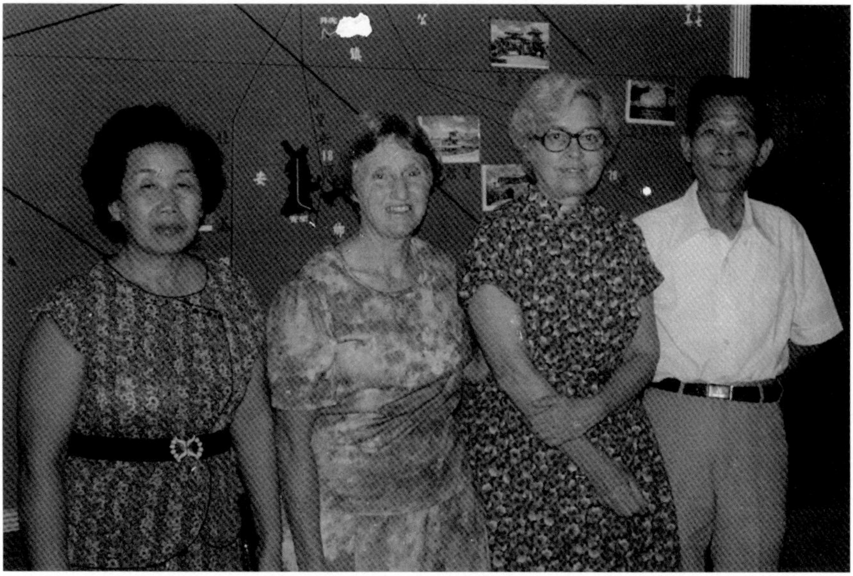

Mrs Whang, Anne Walker, Marjorie Bly, and paramedical worker Stephen - Pescadores, Taiwan

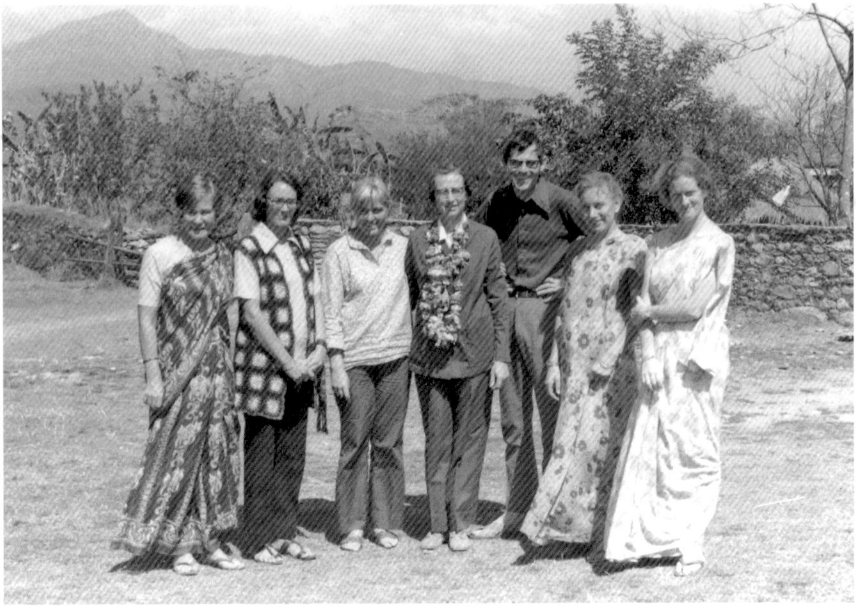

Staff at Pokhara, including Dr Paul Kaltoff and Jeanette Highland (second from left) farewell Dr Grace - Nepal

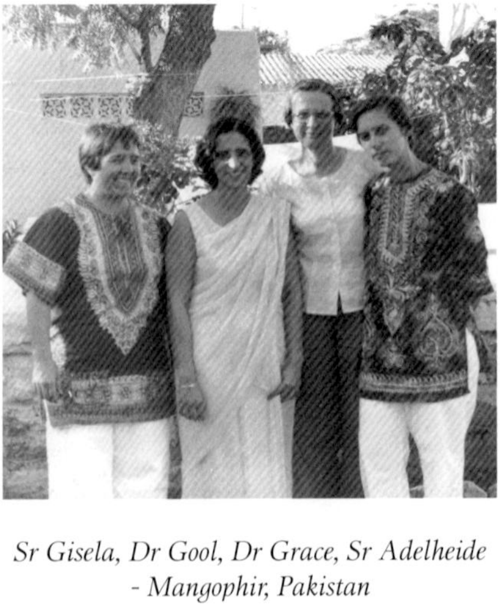

Sr Gisela, Dr Gool, Dr Grace, Sr Adelheide - Mangophir, Pakistan

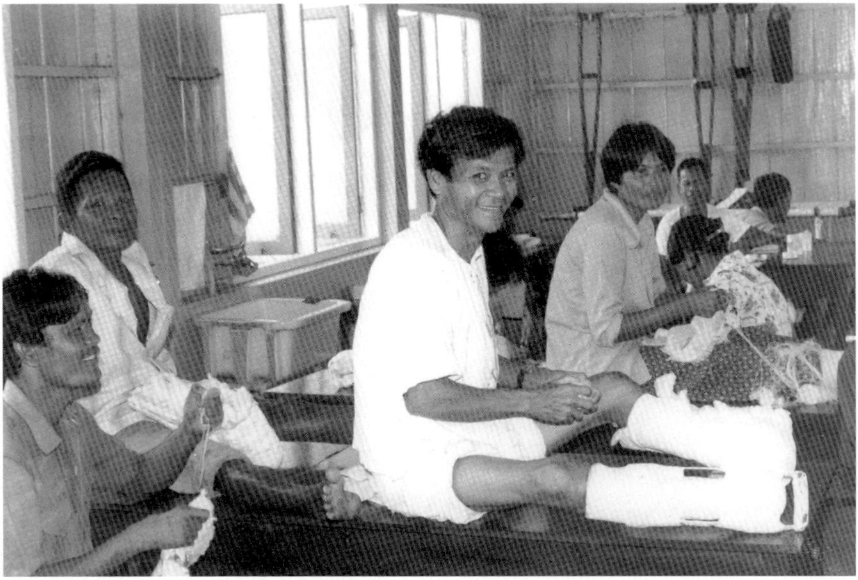

Patients doing physiotherapy - Manorom, Thailand

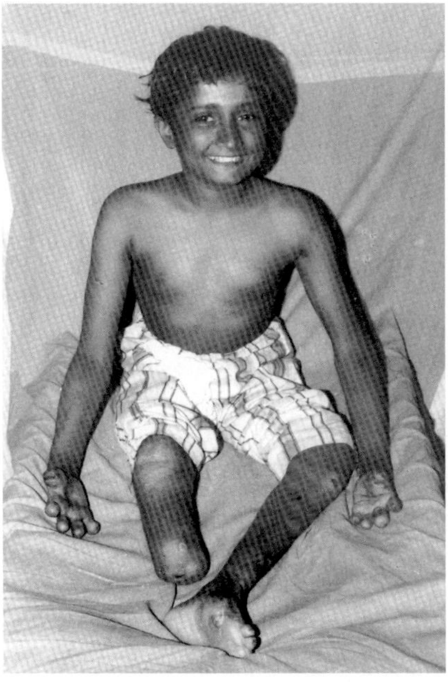

Young boy Sali (short fingers, loss of right leg & abnormality of toes on left foot) – Mangophir, Pakistan 1975

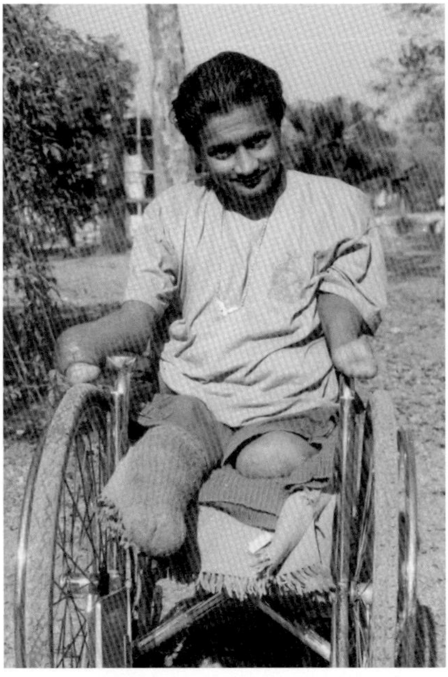

Adult Sali (hands and legs worn away! But no pain, happy, and runs family business) - Rawalpindi 2000

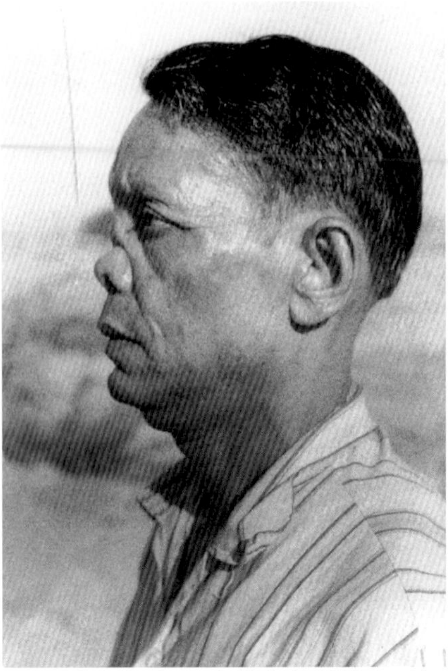

Man in Pakistan with typical leprosy nose deformity

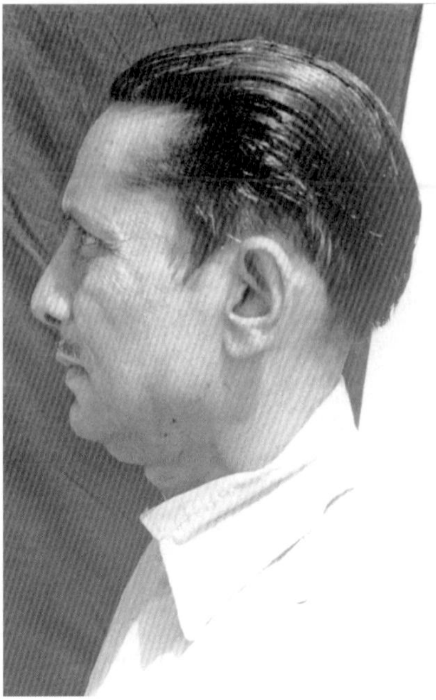

Post operative view of nose after reconstruction

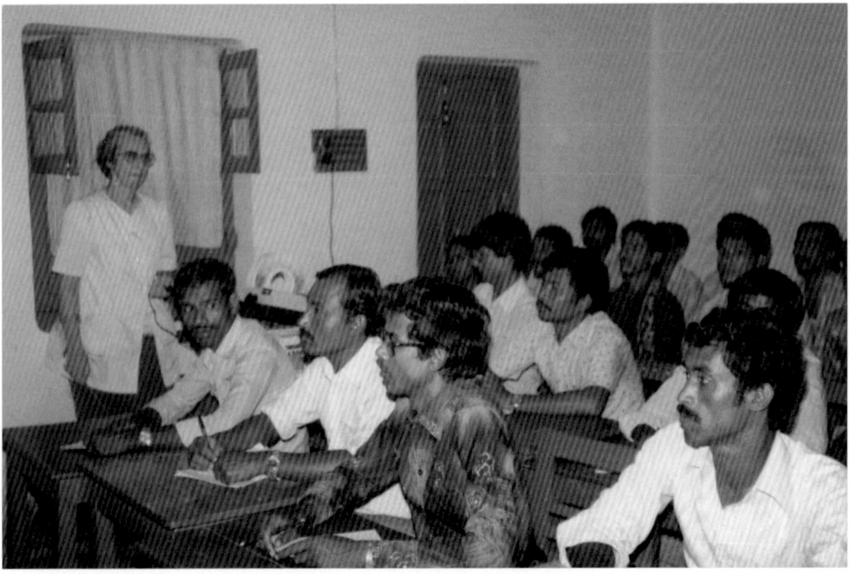

Dr Grace lecturing in Bangladesh

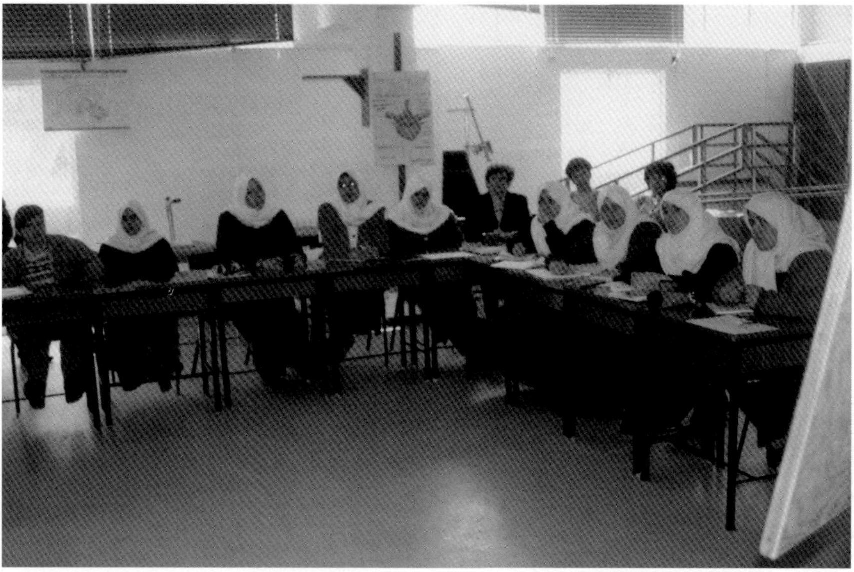

Lecturing physiotherapy students - West Bank, Israel

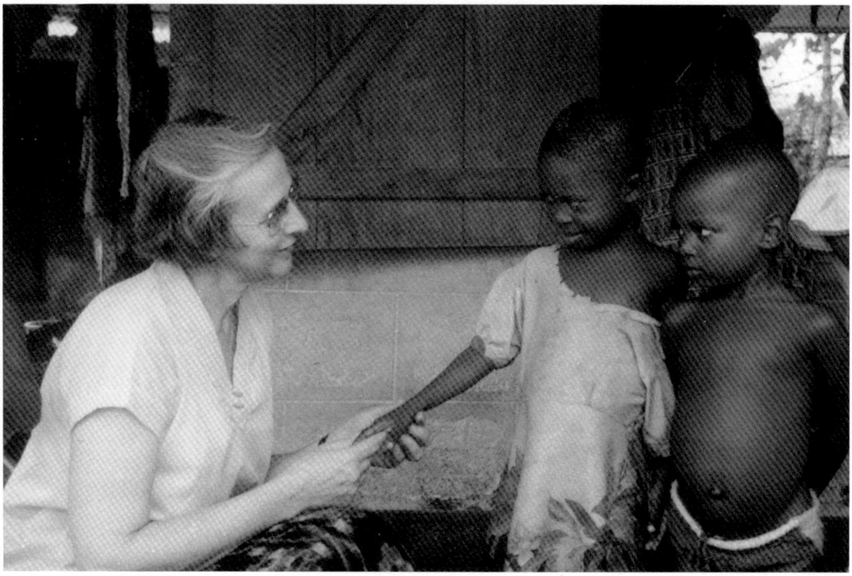

Making friends in Nigeria

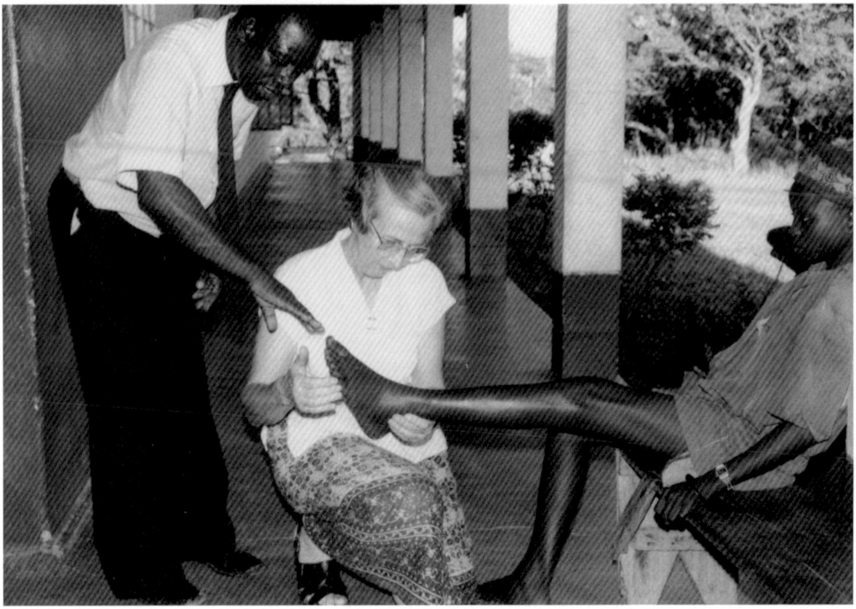

Dr Grace examines a foot in Nigeria

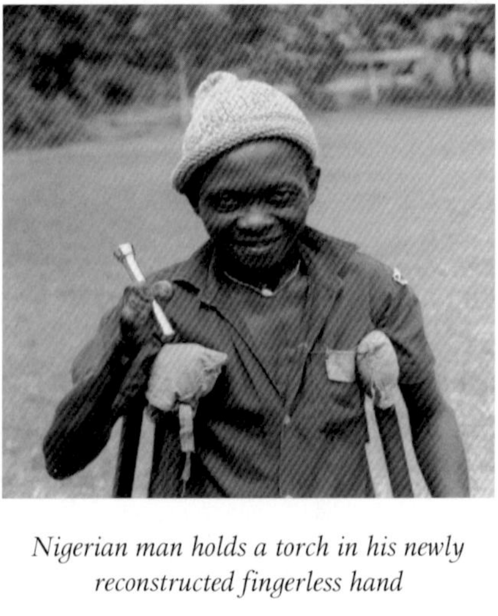

Nigerian man holds a torch in his newly reconstructed fingerless hand

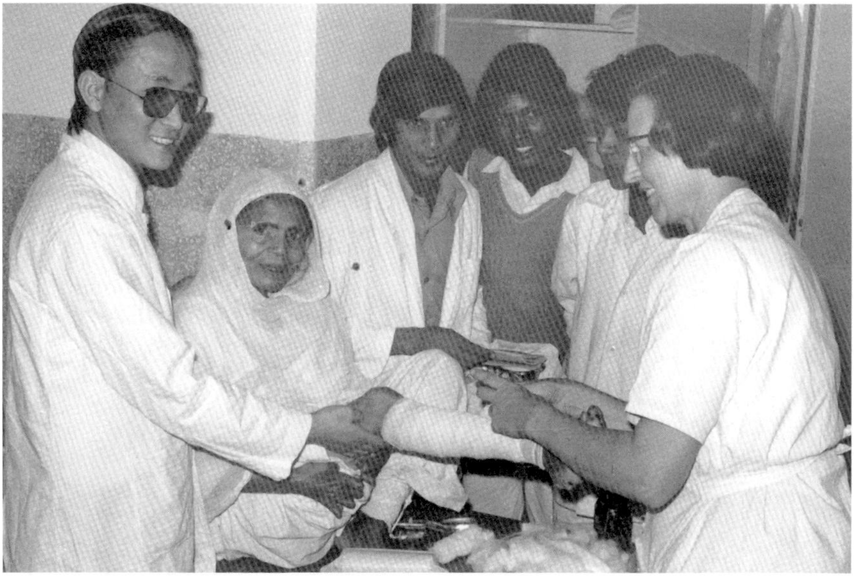

Dr Thomas Chiang learning to apply plaster casts - Karachi, Pakistan

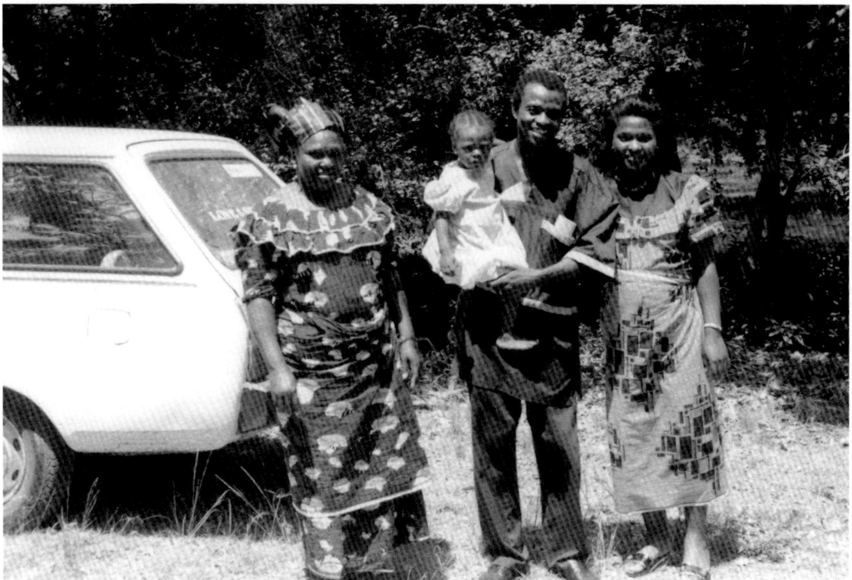

Dr Osahom Ogbewei with his wife Grace and daughter - Ebe, Nigeria

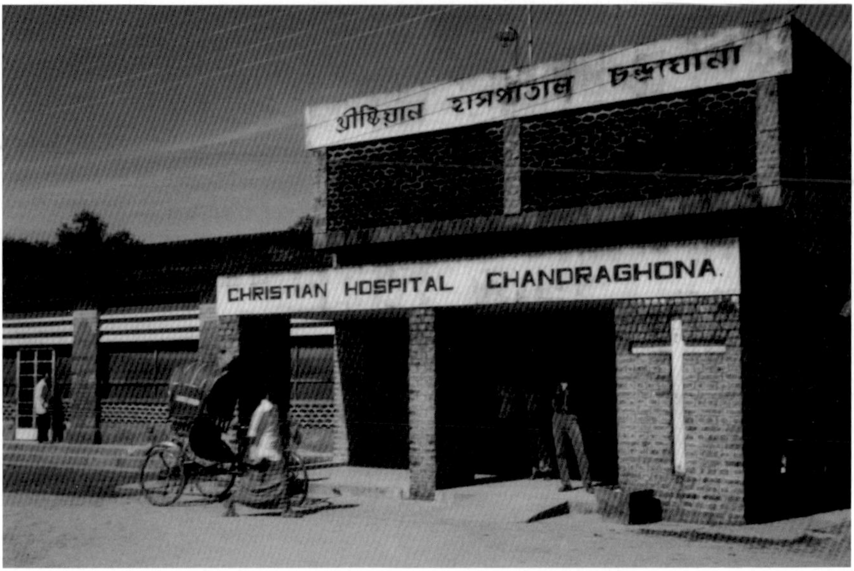

Entrance to Christian Hospital in Chandraghona, Bangladesh

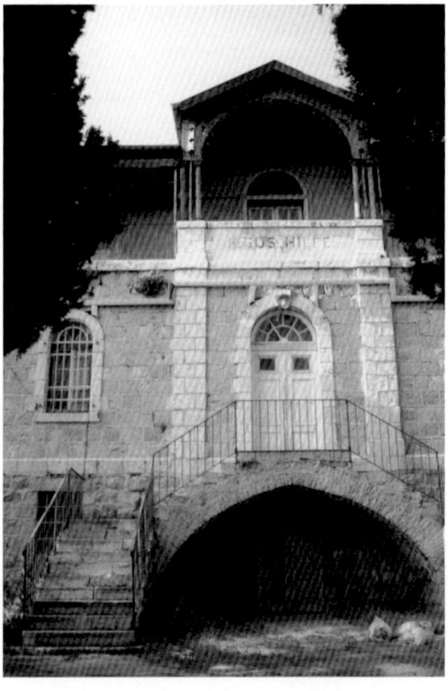

The old main entrance to the leprosy hospital in Jerusalem. "Jesus Helps" is written in German over the entrance

makers. Out of hours he has asked me to see people who had physiotherapy problems and has taken me to their homes. He is what Christians call a "second mile person" (from a saying of Jesus in his Sermon on the Mount) – one who goes much further than the minimum to give needed help.

Since about 2000, Mr Somkiet has been working on Saturdays in a big private hospital which does a lot of diabetic foot care. So he asked me to attend a clinic at this hospital. I had a very warm welcome. We spent the morning at the Outpatients' Clinic seeing the patients. He'd arranged for several people with problem feet to come in for me to discuss their management with the doctors in charge, followed by an afternoon 'seminar' in which patients and their problems were presented. I discussed with staff members what I would do for the particular patients. I know I am welcome there whenever I have time in Bangkok.

Somkiet introduced me to one patient – not with leprosy – who had suffered an unusual accident to one leg. He walked with a foot-drop somewhat similar to that of leprosy patients. He had been to various specialists in Bangkok without any adequate solution to his problem and ended up seeing Mr Somkiat, who got me involved.

Since I was just leaving Bangkok, I sent him off with a letter to OMF's Dr Scott Murray, who does the leprosy work at the Manorom Christian Hospital. It was some time later that I learned that Scott had operated on him. He had done a tendon transfer and some bone surgery to reshape the deformed foot. The man was now walking in a basically normal way and was so grateful. Previously he had been given so very little hope. His problems were not the regular sort of ones which are described in the orthopaedic text books. Too often students are taught by rote what to do for this or that problem. They may not learn how to think around an unusual problem and come up with a practical answer.

A non-leprosy patient at Chiang Mai posed similar challenges. He was an adult when a coconut palm fell on him and broke his back. Johnny had spent months lying on a wooden floor and had huge pressure sores over his buttocks.

He was sent to McKean by missionaries who found him. We applied skin grafts and eventually Johnny's backside was completely healed. With a degree of recovery, the question was: "What could Johnny do?" There was no way he could go back to the mountains. The artificial limb makers at Chiang Mai made him a long pair of metal calipers so he could stand. There were hinges in the knees, so that he could bend them to sit down. He moved around the hospital in a wheelchair – and he wanted something to do to keep himself occupied.

Johnny got a job in the lacquer shop. Because he could stand upright in these calipers, he had a job washing the lacquer-ware. He became a central part of the lacquer-ware team, which produces some beautiful work.

A lot of this sort of work by patients went on at McKean. Since few have had any formal education, it would be virtually impossible for them to get a job in an office, or something similar, in or near their own homes. But as part of a team in Chiang Mai, working together with others, they are able to produce some very beautiful and useful pieces of handwork.

One dear old man with very bad hands needed to be occupied. Heather Smith, an Australian, the wife of Dr Trevor Smith, came up with a way that, even with those hands, he could make Christmas cards, using a type of stencil and spattering paint to create a picture. These "spatter cards" looked very effective. One day Heather Smith came bustling into the room where he was working. "How many pictures have you got? How much have you got in stock?" He showed her and she said, "Well, I've just received an order – I want 500 cards for sale in Australia!" The old man looked at her and said, "Do you mean to say that people will **buy** the work that I am doing?"

She had given him standing in life. He was producing something that other people wanted and so felt his life was worthwhile. In spite of his deformed hands, feet and face, he could still produce cards which were attractive and appreciated. This is what a lot of our rehabilitation work was about – helping these patients to realise they need not be outcasts. They were still worthwhile people if they were prepared to do what they could for themselves and train to do work that was useful to others.

At Phrapradaeng, there was not much in the way of organised handcraft and some patients were actually able to go out to proper jobs outside the hospital. At Manorom Hospital the patients were taught how to do handcraft that they could do at home, and to bring the finished goods back the next time they came to the clinic. They would then get paid for the work and obtain more supplies to continue. We never want to make the patients dependent on us for the rest of their lives. We want to help them to become independent.

My job as surgeon was to try and reduce the disabilities and the deformities so that they are better able to work and to look after themselves. The physiotherapists help by teaching them how to use their reconstructed limbs and how to protect themselves from damage. The social workers check up on their home situation: where they live and what else they need, such as housing and access to schooling for their children. TLM is a whole team working together to help bring about a better quality of life.

One of the rehabilitation projects at Manorom was organised by TLM worker Alan Davis. Alan used to go out and visit the patients' homes and find out just what they could do. Quite often he would provide them with a pig or two, or a sow that was already pregnant. Piglets went back to Alan to go to someone else, or were sold and the money given back. Pork was very popular – particularly amongst the Chinese. So pig-raising was an excellent industry. Another one was ducks. If the patient's home had an adequate water supply, they might be given a number of ducks to raise; duck is a much prized food, particularly for feasts. In some countries, and to a certain extent Thailand, the livestock in these programs extended to goats or cattle. So animal husbandry became one of the ways by which disabled people could earn a living.

Tailoring was another specialty. If we could provide patients with a sewing machine, they could work in their own homes, particularly if they had had some experience with it before.

At Bangkla, east-north-east of Bangkok, was a good general hospital run by the American Southern Baptist Mission. On the staff was an American surgeon, Al Hood, who was prepared to tackle anything and everything, and at times we worked together. The first time I met him at Bangkla, I arrived mid-morning and had lunch at the hospital while he went home. As he arrived home one of his four kids called out, "What's she like?"

His reply: "She does not look a day over 80!" Al was good fun.

The leprosy patients had their own quarters at the back of the hospital, where those who needed to could live and attend Outpatients every day for treatment, dressings or physiotherapy. A nice young Thai woman doctor, Dr Somphorn, worked with Al Hood at the hospital, and she was keen to learn what she could of leprosy. So when I went we would usually do the medical treatments together.

Dr Somphorn became very good at re-educating muscles. They did not have a proper physiotherapist, so when we did surgery, I would go back at the right time and work with this doctor. If we had operated on a foot I would take the cast off and then teach her how to do the re-education work so that the patient could learn to walk properly.

I made regular trips to Bangkla over about fifteen years. After 1975 I went there regularly to set up a program of surgery for the patients who were under treatment at their clinics. Sometimes I went to their outpatient clinic twenty kilometres away and saw the patients there in order to recommend who should come for treatment. This was a general medical clinic, a good system – patients did not mind going there for treatment as it did not advertise that leprosy was their problem.

The Thai staff at Bangkla were very helpful in the leprosy program. Gradually, over the years, we realised there were fewer and fewer new patients. Eventually the residential hostel at the back of the hospital for leprosy patients was closed and leprosy was fully integrated into the services of Bangkla Hospital.

I have written at length about Thailand, because that was the base from which I worked in many other countries and much of what I learned there I was able to apply elsewhere. By the mid-70s there was a program in action which could be used as a model for others.

25

African Episodes

Africa looks a huge continent on the map. While I felt drawn to many other countries, the only thing that I was really interested in seeing in Africa was the huge Zambezi Falls, and that is what I never did get to see. I had criss-crossed Asia many times and been to Europe but had never got to Africa.

When, in the middle of the 1970s, a letter came asking me if I would be prepared to go to Libya to review the leprosy work and the potential there for reconstructive surgery, I had no good reason not to go.

I had to go via Delhi to get a Libyan visa, then fly to Rome to catch a plane to Libya's capital Tripoli. At the Tripoli airport I scarcely changed any money; as the guest of the Libyan government, with all expenses paid, I could see little need for cash.

Libya is of course, a very male-dominated society. In fact it was a wonder that they were prepared to have a woman come as a consultant. From my hotel I was taken everywhere, usually by the men in their own cars, or in government cars. This was just as well, because on the few occasions I ventured outside the hotel by myself, even though I wore a sort of pseudo-Islamic garb I still felt out of place, as if everyone was watching me. I never felt free to do as I pleased. Even to take photos seemed taboo. I'd heard tales of people having their cameras confiscated and smashed, so I was rather careful what I did with my camera.

I was taken to quite a number of areas, around Tripoli, of course, and Ghazi, the next biggest city, and to some of the outlying clinics. Even then Libya was oil-rich. The leprosy patients were literally paid to attend the clinics and all their travel expenses were met; wages lost were refunded, so there was little excuse not to come.

Actually there were not many patients – only a few hundred in the whole of the country. But no-one was doing reconstructive surgery and it did not seem that anyone was really interested in doing any. Nevertheless, I spent a couple of weeks there, talking and discussing, and then had to write a long report which I duly sent in. I do not think I heard another thing from them – So much for Libya!

Then, in the mid-80s, I was asked if I would go to Nigeria. A New Zealander, Dr Dion Warren, had worked overseas as a younger man and had then gone back to New Zealand to raise his family. Now he was once again working with TLM, in Nigeria. He worked at Ekpene Obom, which was half way between Lagos, the capital, and Calabar, where the famous missionary Mary Slessor from Scotland, had worked in the 1800s. There is now a big medical school at Calabar. Ekpene Obom is a large hospital, part of it general and part leprosy, basically staffed by Nigerians. Dion and his wife Pat, lived and worked there, together with a European physiotherapist. Dion had asked if someone could come; I am not sure if he had asked for me specifically by name, but the mission dobbed me in to help with some of the surgery and to give him some ideas of ways to cope with the job.

In 1988 I flew in to Lagos, where I stayed at a mission guest house overnight, and next day I caught a small plane from Lagos to Harcourt, the nearest airport to Ekpene Obom in the Cross River State. Here Dion Warren picked me up by car, and took me to the huge sprawling hospital, built by missionaries many years ago. It served a very large area, mainly forest.

I have memories of one night when Dion, the physiotherapist and I did ward rounds by torch light because the electricity was off. There were all sorts of problems – patients with every imaginable deformity and disability, some due to leprosy, some to other things. Dion Warren had been doing his best to cope with this, and for a time I helped him.

One of the most dramatic patients there was a man who did not have leprosy at all. He'd been admitted to the general hospital some ten years or so earlier with large swollen legs. I do not think there was a proper diagnosis for him. Eventually a lot of the swelling of the legs went down, but he was left with multiple ulcerations on the tops of his feet (the dorsum) but the soles were quite sound. Nothing they did would make those ulcers heal. They dressed them, splinted them and tried skin grafting many times, but they would not heal.

So Dion asked me what I would do. By then the long bones of the toes were infected. So I suggested that we remove the infected bones and re-shape what was left. I carefully did so, leaving as much skin as I could, enough to cover the top of his foot, the dorsum, with the skin of the sole of his foot. There was no trouble in getting it to heal. It healed straight away. A week later we did the other foot, by which time I was nearly due to leave.

I heard later from Dion that within eight weeks he was walking round in a pair of new shoes and off home. First time he'd been out of that hospital for ten years! That taught me a lovely lesson about blood supply in feet. Many clinicians depend on Doppler readings to assess blood supply. I get criticized because I take a lot of notice of "capillary return". This is the rate at which the colour returns to the tip of the toe after compression. It shows what the patient's blood supply can actually do.

There was a young girl whose hands and feet were badly affected by leprosy and for whom we did several procedures in one go. I have become well known for doing two or three things at once. Well, why not, if you have got the time to do it? It means that patients have one anaesthetic, one lot of antibiotics and have to stay in hospital only once for the surgery. You save everybody time, money and expense. So when there is no risk I do as much as I can in one operating session. It saves calling the same patient back for another session later on.

I remember one little Nigerian man who came to see me because he had no fingers on either hand and had great trouble doing anything for himself. [photo] Dion Warren was intrigued to see my approach to that. As I explained in Chapter 8 (Mr Lum) when a patient loses all his fingers he still has the long bones in the hand, and we can take out the second one to provide a type of lobster claw or pincer hand. It's amazing how much patients can do when we give them a "lobster claw" hand. Although far from beautiful, to create such a hand is a real salvage procedure. In most third world countries, of course, there is no chance of getting a proper artificial arm. Actually, in many cases, lobster claw hands work better, especially if they have some sensation in them and patients can feel something of what they are doing.

Undoubtedly, medically and surgically, Nigeria was fascinating for me.

One of the highlights was a trip to Calabar. There is still a mission station there which is a memorial to Mary Slessor, with a medical college and medical school. I was asked to speak to the staff and students. One day we drove there – and had to stay overnight. It's hard to know what to say about a hospital like that. It was a very big rambling place that had grown, like Topsy, over the years. While it dealt with everything, you would not class it with a large hospital of the same number of beds in developed countries. A lot of things were still very primitive, and many of the senior staff lacked the experience they needed to tackle all their problems. I did some lecturing. I tried to teach them a bit about how to assess and deal with the needs of leprosy patients.

In 1989 I travelled to the country next door, Cameroon. This had originally been a German colony, but after World War I it was divided between France and Britain, and now it is part of the United Republic of Cameroon. Up in the hills, in the northern half of the country, is a hospital at Mbingo, run very efficiently by the

American Baptists. Part of that is a special leprosy hospital. The leprosy patients are well treated, with the advantage of American surgeons to operate and help them. I did quite a lot of surgery there. It was interesting working with them, discussing their problems. Many patients needed to live at the hospital for prolonged periods.

The hospital has a wheelchair manufacturing shop. An Englishman had taught the people to make wheelchairs, and they now do them for all over the country. I tried to help them to understand that many leprosy patients, paraplegics and other patients with spinal trauma have no feeling in their buttocks, just where they sit down, and that the hard seating of a chair is not suitable for them. There is a cheap solution – old inner bicycle tubes tied together into a square and pumped up with water make an excellent water cushion, which is much better for the patient with no sensation where he sits down.

While I was there, there was a lively Harvest Festival service on at the local church, with all the women and children singing and chanting. They brought what they had, including live chickens and goats, to the church for the service. It was great fun. The American Baptist couple in charge were lovely people with whom I kept in contact for many years.

I met a young fellow there with many deformities. There was no way we could do all his surgery for him on that trip, and the surgeons at Mbingo felt they could not cope with it all. So on that particular trip we operated on both his feet, doing procedures which the Mbingo surgeons were interested in learning how to do. The following year when I went back to Nigeria he came across the border to Ekpene Obom Hospital and I was able to do some more surgery for him, to his hands. He was a well-educated intelligent young man of about 20, so I do hope that he has been able to make the most of what we did for him.

When I was leaving Mbingo the patients presented me with a

beautiful drip-dry tablecloth – never needs ironing – embroidered with Christmas motifs of red poinsettias and green leaves – a beautiful thing that gives me great pleasure; it has had pride of place for my Christmas table ever since. The patients do a lot of handwork and handcraft and they obviously appreciated what I could do to help them.

In 1990 I went back to Ekpene Obom. I flew into Lagos and again had to stay overnight. Then I was told that something was wrong with the flights so I had to get to a particular town by taxi. I was given the address. I guess there are not too many Western women who would take a six or seven hundred kilometre taxi ride across an unknown tropical country to reach a leprosy hospital near a distant township! The taxi had multiple hiring so four of us started off. I was the one who had furthest to go. That was quite an entertainment! My taxi was eventually met by Dion for the rest of the trip to the hospital.

There I discovered that many patients were not actually getting multi-drug therapy (MDT) even though WHO was recommending it by then. I was discussing it with one of the African doctors, who said: "Oh, well, there are lots of leprosy patients around out in the forest." So I said: "Why do not you go and get them and bring them in and get them treated?"

"Oh" he said "we haven't got enough money for that. We've only got a certain amount of leprosy drugs and we could not possibly treat all the people around here who need to have treatment."

That was the situation in so many of these places. The patients did not get treatment because there just was not enough money to provide it for everybody in that particular community. Unaided, third world countries cannot afford leprosy medicine. Moreover, there are patients who do not complete their courses, and end up with resistance to the medicines we use to kill the organisms causing leprosy. That becomes a real problem,a tragedy for them. TLM provides anti-leprosy medication free to other groups when we feel it is needed. As usual, patients had not been taught how to look after their ulcers. So I was off again on my hobby horse, trying to teach the patients to prevent ulcers or to give them a chance to heal.

Leprosy was or is extremely common in Nigeria. It was said to have one of the highest incidences of leprosy in the world. In Dr Stanley Browne's days, the 1950s and early 1960s, a very high proportion of the leprosy patients were under regular treatment. But internal strife, coups, inter-tribal fighting and the rest had devastated the health system. When I was there, hundreds, if not thousands of patients were not being treated. Nobody knew where they were. A lot of the records had been lost. That is the sort of problem that the World Health Organisation is up against in its campaign "to eliminate leprosy as a public health problem by the year 2010." Nigeria still has huge leprosy problems.

Dion Warren and I again worked together for a short time in Ekpene Obom. I then travelled with him and his wife, Pat, by car up into the hills to a hospital at a place called Ebe – again a very good hospital. It had been built by Presbyterian missionaries and was still partly maintained by them, though mainly staffed by nationals. In charge of the leprosy program at Ebe was Dr Osahom Ogbewei, and his charming wife, Grace. I had met them on my first trip to Ekpene Obom where Osahom was learning leprosy. He has remained with the Mission and now holds an important senior job. Surgeons in the hospital at Ebe were very keen to learn rehabilitation surgery, so we did quite a lot of surgical work there.

That was my last work trip to Africa. Since that time I've only flown in and out of Cairo.

26

Singapore and Conferences

In May 1976, I was in Singapore again to take part in the Pan Pacific Conference of the Society for Rehabilitation of the Disabled – a useful talkfest held every three years. I had been at these conferences in Manila in 1962, Tokyo 1965, Hong Kong 1968, and in Australia in 1972.

As usual, there was also surgery to be done. Things had changed greatly since my many earlier visits. The Trafalgar Hospital which had once been only for leprosy, was now considerably smaller, housing a number of permanently disabled patients needing care. The government orthopaedic surgeons were still prepared to do the reconstructive surgery that we felt would benefit the patients under our care. Patients who needed full medical care and reconstructive surgery, were admitted to Tan Tock Seng Hospital and were cared for in the ordinary wards.

After having worked with about eight or ten doctors for a decade from the mid-1960s, I now came to be working with just one doctor – Dr Lo, an orthopaedic surgeon. He was very pleased to learn what he could from me regarding leprosy management.

Whenever I visited Singapore, Dr Tulip Tan, who had become head of the Leprosy Division, would ask me to lecture the doctors working in the Dermatology Department, which looked after leprosy in Singapore. Singapore had had an effective system ever since the 1950s, whereby every school child was checked for leprosy or any other skin disease at least twice during school years, as a small child and then again as a teenager. Their skin was checked for patches and nerves were palpated. Under the general umbrella of dermatology, if anything showed up, the child would be further investigated and his family at home would also be checked to see if others had the disease. This program made it quite easy to pick up leprosy cases along with psoriasis and other skin problems, without having people incur the feared leprosy stigma. They were just referred to the Dermatological Institute and were dealt with there, just as if they had any other skin condition.

So, in the seventies, Singapore was well ahead in the management of leprosy. They had been using dapsone since at least the early 1950s. Yet, even after 20 years of treatment and school surveys and following up the family contacts, they were still diagnosing several hundred every year. Singapore's population was only about two million in the 1960/70s, but at that stage the percentage of leprosy cases was quite significant.

Singapore has a mixture of races – Chinese, Malays and Indians are the three dominant groups. Those of Indian background had the largest proportion of leprosy patients, though the Chinese, the major population group, had the biggest actual number of leprosy cases, and had the greatest fear of the disease. Nevertheless Singapore has continued to be one of the most advanced places in leprosy care, and now fewer and fewer cases are occurring. Most newly diagnosed cases are "imports" from neighbouring countries.

At the Pan Pacific conference, I had the job of organising the leprosy section and reading a paper on aspects of surgery. I called it "Mind Those Looks". This was deliberately ambiguous. It referred firstly to the visual aspects of leprosy – how to help a patient to be socially acceptable by surgically correcting deformities and disabilities – and secondly to the need for compassionate and non-discriminatory ways of looking at and caring for people who had often suffered such tragic social rejection.

As I was setting up, an elderly gentleman wandered into the room and peered around. I asked if he were looking for something. "Yes" he replied "and you're it." He was Dr Guy Pulvertaft, a retired but active senior hand surgeon from UK, who was conducting a training course in surgery in Singapore. He had been advised to look me up by a colleague who had worked with me in Hong Kong. We became friends, and he invited me to attend his lectures and demonstrations whenever I was free, and I took as much advantage of that as possible. It made for a very busy week! I learnt from him a few more of his techniques, such as how he weaves tendons together in a "Pulvertaft join". I regularly use that when I am joining tendons, particularly on the foot. Later, in the UK I was able to contact him and discuss things with him in order to find the best solution for some problem hands.

About the same time as this general conference there was a TLM conference. It provided an excellent chance to discuss, with surgeons like Paul Brand and Ernest Fritschi, where leprosy surgery was heading, and to talk with the director, Eddie Askew, and board members about changing Mission policies and adaptations to the WHO recommendations regarding treatment. A number of Indian workers with the mission were able to attend – but only if they did not take any rupees out of India. So TLM had to provide all their expenses including some spending money!

There were times of real Christian fellowship and teaching as well as the more work-orientated sessions. There was some hilarity too. One of the German delegates got up one day to have a bit of fun and talked about staining the leprosy bacillus *in situ* – meaning in the patient! The leprosy bacillus is a difficult one to stain and you use a very strong red stain. Then you soak the specimen in alcohol to remove the stain from everything else except the leprosy bacillus. So we got some good laughs as he talked about staining patients and soaking them in alcohol!

It was the first time I had been to one of these big TLM conferences. On this occasion it was held in the 'field', and included both people from the sending countries and the workers from the countries in which we were serving. It was very worthwhile. Discussion groups included dealing with hypothetical applicants to the mission for overseas service – how we would deal with particular people and whether we would accept them in the mission. Those sorts of things I found very helpful. Working as we were without a lot of contact with people from TLM headquarters, we often found it difficult to know why the mission makes the decisions it does. We needed to know where the mission stood on difficult issues.

People often volunteer to come and work in mission situations without any real concept of the background and needs of the cultural group we are serving. Young people in Western countries, even those sent by churches, often have very different ethical and moral standards from those of forty years ago. Today some think nothing of going abroad with a partner of the opposite sex and rooming together even though not married. But in other cultures this may not be acceptable. On one occasion, a young couple arrived expecting to share a room, and the receiving group were shocked to find that they were not married. In another place, a couple turned up who were close friends – they did marry the following year. In that culture however, cohabitation was absolutely out – virtually a capital offence! They had to have separate rooms – and in this case they did oblige. Many of our friends at home, who are happy to support us in our work, do not realise the issues and problems that we encounter in everyday life abroad.

My medical knowledge of Singapore was very useful. One evening one of our delegates, an older man, tripped on the step into the bathroom and fell and broke his nose. We had lots of doctors but no instruments! So I phoned a surgeon I knew, who arranged for us to borrow an appropriate set from a local private hospital. It was rather a hoot; Dr Grace organised with a gynaecologist to get the instruments to reset the broken nose of an elderly leprosy conference delegate! We provided first aid for him in his hotel room.

Later in 1976, I was able to come to Australia for a short leave, as there were quite a few matters at home which required my attention. I called at Sydney University, and Professor John Lowenthal, the Professor of Surgery who had accepted my Master of Surgery thesis, invited me to become a guest lecturer when it was convenient. His offer sounded very interesting because it would allow me to do some extra study and research at the university, and also to teach the students something of what I knew of neuropathy, and to rub shoulders with some of my surgical colleagues. We tentatively arranged for three months in 1979.

Then I went back to Hong Kong, Taiwan and Korea. I had not been into Korea for about seven years, and I wondered if I would remember any Korean language. I did manage to find my own way from the airport by taxi to the recently opened new bus station. That did require some Korean, which just came back to me whilst I was sitting in the taxi! I arrived at Taegu by bus to be met by Grace Bennett, TLM nurse from the UK.

Each year from 1965 to 1968 I had visited the mission hospital in the grounds of the University Medical School. Later, TLM constructed a new four-storey clinic block, with all necessary facilities and a waiting room big enough for a Bible woman to conduct morning services and to teach patients as they waited to be seen.

Dr Kim Mahali was well established as a dermatologist, but spent most of her time doing outpatient clinics. A mobile clinic served leprosy villages and other smaller clinics, dealing with all kinds of skin ailments. Dr Kim was a lovely girl. She had become a Christian while she was working with us, and she really shone with the love of Jesus in the way she treated the patients and dealt with their problems.

Several patients who did not have leprosy came through the

Taegu hospital. I was able to do some serial operations, and the university doctors operated there also. We were able to help one boy had very bad burn scars on his face. Quite a number of patients had facial muscles paralysed due to leprosy, and there was the constant run of hand and foot problems.

I had seen one man, Ee-See, first as a youth in the 1960s. He had mild leprosy, but had to use crutches as he had a terrible pair of feet unable to take his weight. We discovered that he had spina bifida, and had never gone to school. Then he developed leprosy and was brought to our hospital.

Well, throw me a challenge like a really funny pair of feet and I need to find an answer. We X-rayed Ee-See's feet and his spine so we knew exactly what the primary pathology causing the nerve problems. We then operated over a period of several years, first on one foot and then on the other. Eventually his feet were stable enough to take his weight, though with a wide stance because he had lost his sense of balance. By the 1970s, Ee-See had not only learnt to walk, but had become a dare-devil bikie, roaring around on a motor bike making a nuisance of himself – so that I guess some people were sorry that we had patched him up and widened his life options!

A visit to Korea would not have been complete without a quick trip down to Pusan to the Il Sin Hospital where it all started in 1957. There I found a young woman doctor with a badly deformed face due to a connective tissue disorder, not leprosy. I was able to arrange for her to have the special surgery she needed in Australia, free for people from developing countries. The outcome was that she looked much better and literally could show her face to the world again. She returned to the Il Sin Hospital and became one of the senior doctors there. There is no way I could have tackled her needs myself.

27

FRACS AND THEREAFTER

In September 1977, I was again heading home. The highlight of that time was the presentation to me in Canberra of the Fellowship of the Royal Australasian College of Surgeons. It was at a scientific meeting with papers to be read and heard and displays of medical products during the day sessions. But Friday night was my big night.

The College had a number of other presentations to make, and they had arranged that the Friday evening would be a special evening with a buffet supper after the meeting, when I would receive the Fellowship and the others, their awards. But I would also be asked to present the "The Hamilton Russell Memorial Oration", named in honour of one of Australia's pioneer surgeons. Hamilton Russell was part of the group that established the Australasian College of Surgeons as a separate entity, rather than its being just a branch of the English college.

So come the big night I was suitably attired in a lovely full length Thai outfit, burgundy in colour, showing off the gold of the College Gown, with which I would be robed after I had been officially given my Fellowship. I was escorted at the head of a procession of robed dignitaries into the Main Hall and up to the platform by Edward (later Sir Edward) Hughes, who was then President of the Royal Australasian College of Surgeons. The assembled conference delegates stood when we came in. Quite a scene of pomp and ceremony!

After all the presentations and ceremonies, and having received my Fellowship, I delivered the Oration. It was entitled *Peripatetic Leprosy Surgeon.* I was confident that what I had to say would be relevant, as Tom Reeve and I had discussed it beforehand. Tom was then professor of surgery at the Royal North Shore Hospital where once I had been a student. He introduced me and read the citation, which is always read when somebody receives a special award or degree at the College meetings.

Now, "peripatetic" is hardly an everyday term. It derives from the word used to describe the Greek philosopher Aristotle's habit of strolling in the garden as he taught his students. He walked about (Greek *peripatetikos)* as he taught. I loved that title, for I guess that is what I had been doing – and have continued to do over the years: teaching as I travel across Asia. I have been told that I only have to open my mouth and I start teaching. I guess that is inherited from my mother's side of the family. She was a school teacher. My uncle Fred, her brother, was an excellent teacher, and my brother David began his career as a school teacher. I too am a teacher – of sorts.

The lecture, besides presenting the topic of leprosy, enabled me to relate how I got into leprosy work, doing it as a Christian service, because I had done medicine with a view to becoming a missionary. I was also able to bring it right into line with the audience of surgeons, by showing the sort of reconstructive surgery that Paul Brand had developed and popularised, and which by that time was also being applied to diabetes, to post-trauma patients and to others who had problems similar to those of leprosy.

I accented our policy of ensuring that the patient really wanted reconstructive surgery, and was prepared to do his or her part afterwards to re-educate the limb so that it would work well – without which we would be wasting our time. However I also mentioned other procedures more suitable for the feet of 70 and 80-year-olds, that could improve walking without such long hard physiotherapy work for rehabilitation. Few of that age can learn how to automatically use a transferred muscle in a new job. So I conveyed to these surgeons how vital it is to select patients carefully, and to match the procedure to the patient, if one is to obtain good results.

Some must have been very impressed by my lecture, because afterwards most of the medical people who had displays in the hall of instruments, sutures, medications and suchlike, gave me the left-overs to take to my work! Also there were Red Cross people there, and later they offered to send me anything that I could use from their collections of medications, equipment and instruments. The Red Cross ran a wonderful recycling service, since discontinued, of sending to mission hospitals or anywhere needed, surplus medical samples and apparatus being discarded by hospitals as they upgraded.

Normally recipients had to pay transport costs, but the New South Wales Red Cross generously arranged the shipping and sent goods to the Thai Red Cross, who had them delivered to me at Manorom Hospital. I used some at Manorom, but was able to send a lot into Burma, supplying the Leprosy Mission hospital at Moulmein with desperately needed drugs and other medical supplies. (See Chapter 22)

The other interesting outcome was that the RACS gave me a cheque, the profits from that particular conference – a four figure sum which more than paid for one of my trips around Asia. Very welcome indeed! I think that a number of the surgeons there that night would have loved to have been able to have the experiences that I had had. I have found often when I have been speaking that many people are almost jealous of what I have been able to do!

The College requires attendance at some of their conferences in order to continue registration as a surgeon. This of course was the first one I had been to in Australia, now as a newly elected Fellow. The College was really very considerate of my situation. I certainly paid the official fee necessary to be granted the diploma of the College, which gives one the title "Fellow of the Royal Australasian

College of Surgeons" (FRACS) to go after one's name, but as a missionary, I was exempted from the annual subscription. That has continued up to the present – even after I officially retired from TLM overseas work. Since I was continuing to go to Third World countries teaching, and since my work in Australia was mostly teaching too, it was agreed that I should be left as a "missionary", so that I do not get hit with the high fees that surgeons have to pay to keep their name on the Surgical Register. I can also make use of the College library, having articles I needed from reference books sent to me.

I spent a few months at home on that trip as I had other things to do. I remained in Australia till January 1978, so that I could take part in a number of Christian conferences. It was at one of these that we got the devastating news that there had been a road accident just near Manorom Hospital in Thailand. A group of the Manorom staff, OMF missionaries with their children, were driving the hospital mini-bus to a children's celebration, in the neighbouring town of Nakhon Sawan, when another vehicle pulled out sharply from behind a truck and hit them head on, killing 12 people and injuring others. I was the only person in Sydney at the time who knew the people who were in the bus, so I was asked to tell what I knew of each of those involved. Amongst those killed were the wife and two children of Dr Brian Parry, a New Zealander. He was on duty at the hospital, but his wife and their three children were in the bus, and only the eldest boy, Matthew, survived. When the survivors got back to the hospital Brian had to hand his son over to others and concentrate on surgery to save the life of another victim. Our thoughts and prayers were with all the bereaved, mine especially with Brian – what would happen to him now? He had been planning to go to the UK later in the year to complete his surgical training.

I returned to Manorom Hospital in February and was able to help with the rehabilitation of some of those injured. In fact, one woman had a fractured arm that would be very difficult to immobilise. In Sydney I had been able to acquire, free of charge, a suitable metal plate to fix the broken bones together, and at Manorom I assisted Brian Parry in applying it. The result in that case was all we could have asked for.

So I was kept busy until May 1978, when the RACS held its Annual Scientific Meeting, on this occasion offshore in Kuala Lumpur, and I was able to go to that international conference.

Amongst the people there was Mr H. H. Eastcott, a senior vascular surgeon in England. He was the 'boss' of an English surgeon at Manorom who had been killed in the crash. I got to know Mr Eastcott and later met and worked with him in London. He, on his part, wanted to know all about the crash and who else had been killed. So I told him about Brian having lost his wife and children and being hesitant about going to UK that year to do his fellowship of the English College. Mr Eastcott asked me to give Brian a message, that he would help if he could and for Brian to contact him when he got to UK.

Brian did get to UK in 1978 and Mr Eastcott was better than his word. Brian notified him that he had arrived and had applied to go to Bristol for training. But an invitation came from Mr Eastcott to come to his Harley Street rooms for "tea" on a certain afternoon. Now it is said that such an invitation is as binding as a royal invitation! Brian turned up, was introduced to the head of one of the main hospitals in London, who then offered him a training position in his hospital. This was one of the top hospitals where a man from the 'colonies' had little hope of entry! This wonderful job opened the way to other special privileges and Brian had his FRCS in near-record time.

In due course Brian returned to New Zealand, where opportunities opened out because of his ability, his excellent training and achievement of the Fellowship of the Royal College of

Surgeons of Edinburgh; later he gained his FRACS too. Brian is now a professor in surgery in Auckland. He has remarried and has more children. Matthew is, of course, an adult, and the second group of children are grown up too.

It was a real pleasure to work with Brian and he always greets me very warmly when we meet at conferences. So it is another of those stories of how God uses even accidents and tragedies to work things out to his glory. Brian is a very keen supporter of medical mission work in third world countries. He has a basic understanding of leprosy and also appreciates the type of rehabilitation surgery that I do.

For me 1978 was a year of much travel, including Taiwan, Korea and Hong Kong. Then I went to Mexico to attend a Leprosy Congress, via the UK, with a side trip to Northern Ireland for a heavy schedule of TLM deputation meetings.

On one occasion there I was an after dinner speaker. It was my second night in Ireland and I was suffering jet lag. The dinner was late, and when eventually they asked me to speak it was after 11 pm their time, about 9 am Thai time, and long past my bed time! Anyhow the talk proceeded till well after midnight, with questions afterwards. On the way home my host and driver said he'd been fascinated watching me: "You talked about each slide and changed from one to the next and never missed a beat – but when I looked at you I could see that often your eyes were shut and you were swaying on your feet. It looked as if you were asleep!" Well, maybe I was!

This is one of the advantages of giving lectures on topics that one is really familiar with. Slides are most helpful because they act as my notes and my prompts, and in third world countries people can often read English much better than they can understand it as spoken.

I then went back to London to the Hospital for Tropical Diseases and met Michael Waters again. I had worked with Michael on many occasions in the earlier 1970s at Sungei Buloh, Kuala Lumpur. In 1978 he was doing leprosy clinics at the Hospital for Tropical

Diseases, which was affiliated with University College Hospital, London. He arranged for me to see some of his patients. I was able to advise which kind of surgery was needed for each. He did not have anybody readily available in the UK who was familiar with leprosy surgery and able to do it for him.

So he arranged for me to see some patients with a Professor of Surgery at UCH. He in turn brought his registrar, who was in training as a hand surgeon.

There was a particular patient from Pakistan, who had had an accident, causing a characteristic nerve deformity of the little and ring fingers of the left hand. It was a deformity very similar to the ones the leprosy patients develop. The Professor asked the registrar what he would do for the patient. The registrar admitted, "Well sir, nothing – I am not sure I could improve either the function or the appearance of the hand." When the Professor asked me, I told him what I would do. He then requested that I return to UK and work with Michael to teach at UCH, for the benefit of UK patients, the surgery that we had perfected for leprosy. So I visited approximately every two years from that time on.

I was an official delegate at the International Leprosy Congress in Mexico City, and was also taking part in one of the pre-congress workshops. It is quite usual for these international conferences to be preceded by workshops of various different specialties, and I was part of a discussion group on surgery. We spent two days in discussion and then a summary of our findings was presented at the conference. It was so good to be part of a peer group at that time.

A few of us, who had been working together, shared a taxi for some sightseeing. The taxi driver, a Roman Catholic unacquainted with Protestants, was baffled by these very strange foreigners. He could not comprehend that Ernest Fritschi, a surgeon working with us in leprosy and also an ordained minister or priest, could be unabashed about having a wife and children at home!

In medical conferences there can be many hours which can seem wasted. In the leprosy field everybody has their say about whatever they are doing: restorative work, or physiotherapy, or making shoes, or whatever. But often it is the informal encounters and conversations that make the whole thing worthwhile. Having a really good huddle, getting together and discussing our mutual problems outside the official meetings is the best thing about conferences.

It was while I was in Mexico that we had several private discussions about the problems in Nepal. The government in Nepal had requested that more teaching be given for the Nepali staff at all levels, and discussions were under way. Could I be involved in the program to be started in 1979?

28

Bangladesh

I happened to be in Karachi, West Pakistan, in 1971 when the unrest commenced in East Pakistan, leading eventually to its declaration of independence as Bangladesh in 1972. At that time many Hindus living in East Bengal fled to India, and many others, Muslims, living in the eastern state fled as refugees to Karachi. As fellow Muslims, they were accepted as Pakistanis at that time and could get jobs. Dr Thomas Chiang also came as a refugee from war-torn East Pakistan at that time; his story is told in Chapter 10. He worked in Karachi at the Marie Adelaide Centre.

Before this upheaval in the early seventies, the leprosy work in East Pakistan was mainly overseen from Karachi. Paramedical workers were trained in Karachi, and people from the eastern state would come over to work with me there, to learn something about leprosy work in general and reconstructive surgery in particular, so that they could apply it in East Pakistan. After 1972 the Bangladeshis had to go it alone and needed to set up their own leprosy program, with headquarters in the capital, Dhaka. Each of the mission hospitals around Bangladesh had to restructure their leprosy work for the new situation.

I was invited to go to Bangladesh to assist in a course on the treatment and management of leprosy for mission hospitals. When I arrived at Dhaka, in March 1979, I was met by a young Swiss doctor, who had recently done the leprosy course at Karagiri in South India, and was now in charge of the HEED Leprosy Programme at Kamalganj. HEED – Health Education and Economic Development – is a Christian consortium of mission groups, including TLM, who banded together in order to obtain permission from the government to work in Bangladesh, which is of course a Muslim country. The government was not prepared to have Christians running institutions such as schools, but was willing to have people for health and economic development, provided that Christian teaching was not a dominant part of their work. So TLM was one of the organisations that helped to start the Kamalganj HEED Centre east of Dhaka.

On my first trip I was duly taken around the various mission hospitals, so that I could see the problems and gauge what could be done for leprosy patients in Bangladesh. I went the length and breadth of the country: right up into Sylhet in the north-east, way down south-east to the Baptist Hospital in Chittagong, to Rangpur on the north-western side, and lots more in the middle. Then we met in Dhaka for three or four days of teaching, workshops and discussion with an English woman, Dr Margaret Owen, who had been working for many years in Bengal, the Indian state adjacent to Bangladesh. She had good local and cultural knowledge and was most helpful.

It was a very interesting session. Many nationals spoke Hindi as their first language, and the Bengali language, Bangla, as well as English. There were people from all round the world who worked in the various missions, and other volunteer groups which were recognised by the government.

I visited the HEED office several times before the conference, and met a very pleasant local woman who spoke beautiful English. She was not involved in treating leprosy, but she'd heard me chatting and decided she'd like to come to the conference. Afterwards she came up and said "That was fascinating: I could understand you!" That of course was a reflection on the English spoken by other people!

At such a conference I try to avoid Aussie English, with its Australian nasal twang and expressions. I've learnt to speak with a fairly simple vocabulary and a more neutral accent that can be understood internationally. I have found time and again lecturing in these Asian countries that people do understand me. This is shown by the fact that they invite me back! When I am lecturing, I speak slowly. Leprosy expert, Dr Stanley Browne, taught me that, as an international lecturer you should not speak more than one hundred words a minute, which is actually very slow, much slower than the natural rate of Australian, English or American speech. I have trained myself to be able to speak at approximately that rate when necessary.

So, in 1979, began my annual pilgrimage to Bangladesh. I would spend maybe a week at Kamalganj, doing surgery there. Their physiotherapists prepared patients and followed them up. Then I would go on to some of the other centres. We gradually increased the number of places that were doing reconstructive surgery. At the British Baptist Hospital in the south, near Chittagong, a surgeon, Bob Hart, had been doing some reconstructive surgery for years: he thoroughly enjoyed my showing him how to tackle new surgical challenges. Then, in the north-west a year or so later, the Roman Catholic sisters working at a hospital at a place called Dhunjury set up an operating theatre. They were very proud of it when I arrived. They had all the equipment including a big autoclave to sterilize their instruments, but had not a clue how to use it! I had to work out how to operate it. I am grateful for the fact that, as a medical student, I got my fingers into lots of areas besides pure medicine. We got the operation program going and I was able to teach the Italian doctor, Sister Rosa, a nun who had never really done much surgery, how to do some of the simpler procedures. Every year I helped her add to the list of what she could achieve.

Bangladesh has a huge, densely packed population. Nobody knew how many people there were with leprosy. When I first visited, the estimate was 100,000, but there were only about 30,000 on the books. The different non-government organisations were trying to encourage their paramedical workers to go out looking for leprosy sufferers and to bring them in for treatment and care.

Because TLM was one of the approved NGOs, I needed to report to Dr Mohammad Khan, the head of the Government Mycobacterial Services – i.e. all the programs for leprosy and tuberculosis, both of which are caused by a mycobacterium. He and I became quite good friends. We would discuss how best to tackle all sorts of problems and how to get more people involved. The government was working with outpatient clinics rather than hospitalising patients; monitoring was needed to make sure that the patients were getting the right treatment. Each time I visited Bangladesh I would meet him in his office to talk about programs and progress.

One year, in the mid-80s, Dr Khan greeted me in great distress because a colleague had sent a report to the government head office stating, "Now that we have introduced Multi Drug Therapy for our leprosy patients, which only requires 24 doses, the leprosy problems will be overcome in two years. After that we will not require any funding." Dr Khan asked me, "Is this correct?"

I was indignant and emphatic: "Absolutely not! At present you only have about forty thousand patients on your books and yet there are estimates that you may have as many as one hundred thousand patients in Bangladesh! If you start all these forty thousand on MDT, in two years they may have finished treatment, but what about all the others we haven't even found yet? You're not going to find sixty thousand patients and complete their therapy in two years!"

I pointed out that, possibly in two years' time, we might be able to get a large number of these people off the register for active treatment. But by then we should have found many more. "MDT use does not mean that we're not going to need continued services and treatment for people not yet located, not to mention the many more who are incubating the disease without yet showing signs of leprosy."

"'Right," he said, "Will you come to the Ministry of Health and explain it, please?"

The next thing I knew we were whizzing through the back streets of Dhaka. I was ushered in to the Treasurer at the Ministry of Health to explain the difference between our point of view and that of the colleague who was completely mistaken about the ongoing problem of leprosy. This is, of course, one of the big problems with the WHO in its euphoria at the effectiveness of MDT. They want the public to believe that leprosy is being eliminated as a public health problem. They also utterly fail to emphasise the need to prevent and correct deformities.

Groups who are prepared to work in cooperation with the WHO and to give the MDT provided by WHO free or at reduced cost have to meet its criteria for eligibility. But many of the patients who, in my eyes, have obvious leprosy, and who could be proved to have leprosy if adequate biopsies were available, are classified by WHO as **not** having it. But unless those patients are treated now, they are going to become real medical problems in another five or ten years when their disease has spread and become more difficult to treat. We discussed all this with the Ministry of Health Treasurer, and as a result, thankfully, the recommendation made to him to end the WHO support was cancelled.

I had very good cooperation with Dr Khan. He was very helpful as we planned our programs. I discovered from him that the WHO had given large quantities of the drug rifampicin to be used for leprosy patients, but not for tuberculosis. This Rifampicin was sitting in the warehouse on the docks at Chittagong, because the government had not worked out how to distribute it so that it would only go to leprosy and not to tuberculosis (TB) patients. Bangladesh had a very big TB problem, but this rifampicin had been given for leprosy. In the meantime, the drug had passed its use-by date! It seemed then that it was totally useless.

Rifampicin is an expensive drug. Here was a drug that we needed to control leprosy rapidly, and to stop it being spread in the community, and it had sat on the docks going to waste! I managed to get a sample of it to send off to London to Dr Michael Waters at the Hospital for Tropical Diseases. Michael had it examined by the Medical Research Council in England. When the report came back from London it was extremely surprising: although the drug was outdated, its efficacy was in fact ***greater*** than the normal Rifampicin. Some deterioration had occurred, but the actual antibiotic in the capsules was as effective as it would have been if it was new!

With that question settled, the Bangladeshi government set to work to organise getting it out to the NGOs, mostly Christian missions, who were treating leprosy patients, as well as to the government doctors. Hopefully the rifampicin was distributed to the right places before it really did lose its potency. With the authority of the Medical Research Council in England, Dr Mohammad Khan could say that this medicine, although in theory past its use-by date, was in fact quite safe and effective and that no problems should occur from its use to treat leprosy.

For years the government stated that there was no leprosy in the delta area. The great Brahmaputra River flows down from the mountains of Nepal and the Himalayas, and spreads out across the vast flood plain, forming dozens of smaller streams flowing to the sea. The government claimed that there was no leprosy in that area because none were registered for treatment. But at Dhunjury, which was about four hours by train from Khulna, the main city on the delta, the Roman Catholic sisters knew better. They observed that a number of their patients gave addresses from the delta area near Khulna. After a few years of working at Dhunjury, Sister Rosa, who did surgery with me and was one of those in charge of the leprosy program, moved south with some of the other sisters and set up some clinics in the Khulna area. Within a year they literally had hundreds of patients. Of course they had been there all the time, but, as the government did not have a leprosy clinic in the area, they were neglected and undiagnosed.

Another place at which I regularly spoke was the Sylhet Medical College. I happened to know that one of the medical students had leprosy, although few others knew it. So when I was doing my lecturing in my usual way, I threw in the fact that leprosy is probably one of the most infectious diseases that there is. However although it is a most infectious disease, it has an extremely low morbidity. In other words, hundreds of people may catch the disease, but relatively few of them are ever going to show signs of it. "If we do the right sort of tests," I said, "we are able to tell who has had the disease and has cured themselves." So I cast my eyes around the lecture theatre – as I did many times in many places – and asked, "How many of us are here – 400? Well, I'd say that you have probably all caught leprosy because this is an endemic country, but then maybe only twenty of you will ever develop any clinical signs of the disease." You could see them all looking at each other, absolutely horrified. The next thing I threw in was, "But with the modern MDT which the WHO is now recommending, once on treatment a patient rapidly becomes non-infectious, so rapidly that forty-eight hours after the first doses of rifampicin the disease cannot be transmitted to others!" That always astonished the students and stirred their hearts because so many had been brought up to be deeply afraid of leprosy, afraid of what it would do to them and their relatives. The thought that a high proportion of people may have it and that no one ever knows is a scary thing for them. But, of course, if they've had it and cured themselves they are not going to give it to anyone else anyway, so what is the difference! It's very good to throw these sorts of ideas at the students to upset their preconceived ideas of what leprosy is and what can be done for it.

Bangladesh was basically a poor country when I was there, and it still is. It is frequently ravaged by floods, which theoretically could be controlled or at least reduced in severity. It's a fascinating country – a country of great contrasts. The east and central areas grow a lot of tea. Its low foothills are ideal tea territory. When those tea estates were started Indians were brought in as workers. They also brought leprosy with them, so there was a lot of leprosy in the central eastern part of Bangladesh.

TLM had to find somebody else to take over the Kamalganj HEED program when the young Swiss doctor I mentioned left after only one tour of duty. So they asked Ian Cochrane to transfer from Purulia in India.

Ian was virtually of my generation. His father was Dr Robert Cochrane, a great leprosy doctor. Robert wrote one of the most important textbooks on leprosy and had a lot to do with the introduction of dapsone. Ian was born in India, I think, and educated in England where he trained as a doctor. Then he returned to India to work with TLM. Over the years – the 1960s, 70s and 80s – I worked with Ian in a number of places in India, including Karigiri and Vellore. He was assisted by his wife, Marion, who was a nurse, and was able to do a lot to help him remain in his work. Ian not only knew leprosy in the Indian context but also knew the basics of reconstructive surgery.

In Ian's first year there, the number of leprosy patients in the tea estates doubled. This was because he was able to recognise the early signs of leprosy and knew how to manage it. He also did the routine, straightforward reconstructive surgery that he knew he could cope with, and would save for me the complicated, problem cases, or the failed ones that had not worked out. I was able to work with him on these when I next came to Kamalganj. This meant that the whole of the work there was more effective.

That experience with Ian goes to show how important it is to have people in these leprosy programs that really know the disease.

In many countries people are trying to treat leprosy but do not really know enough about it. This means they are probably missing lots of patients and may be mistreating others in whom deformity could be prevented if correct care was given.

I went in and out of Bangladesh for about twelve years: mostly every year, lecturing at most of the medical colleges and leprosy hospitals in the country, as well as to some nursing groups. I had very busy programs around various hospitals doing medical and surgical work. But I haven't been to Bangladesh since the early 1990s. Other people have taken over. Most of the doctors that I was working with have now moved elsewhere, and I am not really in touch with the program now.

I am finding that everywhere I go, not just in Bangladesh, staff need to be much better trained. Everywhere there is the problem of the constant turnover of people working in the leprosy programs. It's encouraging to have young people in Australia, England or USA volunteering to do a year or two, but in such a short period they are only just beginning to get a feel for leprosy and of what can be done for it. Our constant concern is how to get workers to stay longer.

29

Nepal

We visited The Leprosy Mission hospital at Anandaban, Nepal, in 1973 as tourists, but in January 1976 I was asked if I could visit and lend a hand. Dr John Harris had gone to the Congo and Dr Yo Yuasa, the Superintendent, was keen for me to advise and help the Indian surgeon working there, which I did.

It was really wintry. At Anandaban it was lovely to sit by an open fire. The capital Kathmandu is in a valley, quite high in altitude, but Anandaban is a thousand feet higher. Then I flew to Pokhara in another valley, closer to sea level, to visit, for the first time, the Green Pastures Leprosy Hospital operated by the International Nepal Fellowship (INF). The flight was fascinating, with wonderful Himalayan views.

The INF, based in Pokhara, were doing the leprosy work for the central provinces of Nepal at the request of the government, training paramedical workers for their outpatient work of examining, diagnosing and treating patients up in the hills. These young men, who rarely had more than a high school education, were then often posted many days' walk away from supervision. They could always refer anyone back to us at the hospital, but it was obvious that they needed to know how to treat most of the common problems unaided; a man with an infected foot cannot very well be sent to walk three or four days to get to hospital. So the paramedical workers (PMWs) learnt it all, diagnosis and treatment of leprosy, the care of feet, basic ulcer care and the general management of its complications.

I was able to do some lecturing to them, usually through an interpreter, and also to the nursing staff and the other medical personnel, who, even if not directly involved in leprosy work, certainly came up against it in the course of their general medical work.

I worked with a number of doctors there over the years. In those first days in Pokhara it was a German, Dr Paul Kaltoff. He was a very good surgeon and I did some interesting surgery with him. Paul also did some work at the government hospital a couple of kilometres away in the town. I stayed in his house with his wife and children and appreciated being treated as one of the family.

Paul's wife was teaching leprosy patients to do a type of batik painting, and they were selling their products in the Pokhara market to the many tourists who came by on their way to the trekking and mountain climbing. The Annapurna Range dominates the Pokhara Valley and forms the foothills of the mighty Malchapurpra, the Fish Tail Mountain, one of the peaks that people go to Nepal to climb.

The batik project proved so successful that a lot of non-leprosy patients took it up too. At Pokhara there was a great emphasis on handwork, all types of crafts, employments that the patients could follow when they went home. I remember one woman sitting out on the veranda with a foot in a plaster cast, making belts out of local string. She, in turn, was teaching an old man the same craft. The Nepalis wear a type of trouser or a skirt, needing belts to hold them up, so there was always a demand for them. They also did weaving and rug-making, another very popular craft, particularly for people from Tibet. There were many Tibetans in the Pokhara area.

At the Mexico conference, in 1978, the question came up as to whether I might be available to teach a special upgrading course for these paramedical workers and doctors at Pokhara. I was an obvious choice as I'd been there before. Nepal, one of the world's poorest countries, did not have its own medical school at that time, and with leprosy being endemic, it was recognized that the Nepali doctors who had trained elsewhere needed to learn about it. I agreed to go, particularly to teach the surgical side of the course. An English doctor, Dr Harold Wheate, was going to do the bulk of the medical teaching, while some other specialists would be coming from India.

From Mexico I travelled via Japan to Bangkok and then did the usual round of Thai hospitals. Trips to Burma, India and Bangladesh followed before I arrived in Nepal in April 1979.

So began a new phase for me of teaching leprosy. As part of the teaching team, I conducted practical sessions on foot care and also worked with the physiotherapists and others, filling in their medical gaps. I may be known as a surgeon but I started as a leprosy generalist and I still do everything!

I was amazed at the changes at Green Pastures in the few years since I was there before. Staff facilities were now impressive. They frequently held training courses there in various aspects of leprosy care. There was a residential block to accommodate the students, and facilities for meals for about 40-50 students and staff assembled for the course.

The students attending the main course were largely the Nepali doctors trained elsewhere. It was not until the next decade, the eighties, that a full medical course was established in Nepal. All doctors had to speak English, and English text books were generally used, so we could lecture in English, though I had to be careful with my choice of words. Sometimes too, the students used and pronounced words in a surprising manner. Fortunately I had learnt long ago to interpret English as spoken in the Indian sub-continent.

During this visit and several more I made in the eighties I gave further assistance in the training of the INF paramedical workers, who were now being sent, not only to the designated INF areas but all over Nepal. Leprosy is present everywhere but training is only given in the two main centres. I was able to help write a syllabus for the PMW courses, and by so doing, to organize a suitable interpretation and means of applying the new WHO examination and treatment schemes that virtually became a necessity, after 1982, in order to obtain WHO financial assistance.

We were able to devise a program that could enable these men, working in mountain areas many days' walk from the hospital, and lacking modern technology, to diagnose and start patients on correct treatment with reasonable confidence. Of course they did not have the facilities to do a skin smear – that was one of the easier ways of proving that someone had leprosy: finding the leprosy germs in their skin – nor could they do elaborate electrical nerve and muscle testing. They could use their eyes to check the skin and their hands to feel nerves, and they could however ask the patients to do things to check how many muscles were functioning. We were trying to provide training in simple yet reliable ways of properly examining and diagnosing the patients.

One of the people I worked with was Jeanette Highland, who has now gained her doctorate in Public Health and is living back in Tasmania. Jeanette was then very much involved in that training program, and in teaching these workers how to diagnose and treat leprosy, and how to look after the complications that develop.

The WHO provides free medication in countries like Nepal. Its treatment schemes – how much to give, how often and for how long – were mainly based on the number of skin lesions patients had. What I had discovered, and what had not been put into practice in Nepal, was that, in parts of the Indian sub-continent, there were many patients who get what we call Pure Neural Leprosy. The leprosy is in the nerves and these patients suffer nerve damage, but the classical skin lesions are not present. By emphasising skin lesions as a guide to the severity of their leprosy and whether they needed treatment, WHO tended to neglect these patients.

In the late 1970s, we had to work out a system of treatment so that the patients could benefit regardless of the type of leprosy they had. So this was one of the things that I went through with the doctors. We worked out a new regime which simplified matters very much.

I did not visit Nepal again until 1985, when I was asked specifically for my surgical skills and spent some time at both centres. The previous surgeon had left Pokhara and a new one was learning, so I spent some time there teaching surgery and teaching the PMW trainees. Jeanette Highland took me on a trip by car to Tansen Hospital, which is run by the United Mission to Nepal (UMN) and situated south of the mountain chain. To get there from Pokhara one drives along the steep side of a deep gorge through which the Siti River flows, until the road emerges from the mountains and hits the plains to the south; then west across the plain, crossing a number of big rivers, till again the road turns north and climbs up to Tansen in the Himalayan foothills. It was a beautiful drive – prolonged for us because we found one of the big rivers in flash flood, with the road submerged on the top of the dam. We had to sit and wait, with dozens of others, till the water subsided. Once the worst of the rush of water was over, first the buses tested out the causeway. Then, with the buses safely through, the trucks with higher axles followed and then the four-wheel drive vehicles. Fortunately ours was a four-wheel drive so we got through without too much delay.

Tansen Hospital is a general hospital, with expatriate doctors and Nepali people for their other staff, and it has a special leprosy clinic. I was able to help them to find solutions to some of their leprosy medical problems and to give lectures to the leprosy staff. There was a good surgeon there who had not learnt the special surgery for leprosy, so I taught him some of the main operations. Then, on the last day, I operated on his face! He had a partial paralysis that caused him a lot of problems, because he could not shut his right eye: it kept watering and dripping tears – hardly ideal when he was operating! A few years later I again worked with him in Pokhara.

The following year, 1986, I visited Tansen, Pokhara and Anandaban while on my way back from London to Bangkok, setting a pattern of calling in to Nepal every year or two until early in the new century. In the 1980s there was an experienced surgeon at Anandaban, so my visits to teach surgery were not necessary until the early 1990s, when he had returned to Holland, and an Australian, Des Soares, joined the staff and was given the surgeon's job. Des took to the surgery like a duck to water and thoroughly enjoyed my visits, when I could also help him with non-leprosy surgery. Des found that the opportunities at Anandaban enabled him to gain experience for a variety of surgical procedures that he is now able to do in Australia.

It has been fascinating to see the advances in those centres over the years. Pokhara has grown from a pure leprosy hospital to a rehabilitation centre, where a large number of non-leprosy disabled are admitted for treatment. Here expert physiotherapy, with limb and orthotic making, are available, together with the usual supportive measures expected in developed countries. In Nepal, as elsewhere, it is once again the Christian mission hospitals that have set an example, by providing sorely needed care and facilities unavailable in the earlier days in the general medical institutions.

A constant stream of Nepali doctors came to work with us, but did not stay as long as we would have liked them to. However, as they scattered over the country, we trusted that they were taking with them a better understanding of leprosy, and, we hope, of general rehabilitation. There is now a medical college in Pokhara at which I have lectured on a number of occasions. I have also lectured at a new medical college in Kathmandu. Since 2000, Christian missions have also opened a new Leprosy and Rehabilitation Hospital at Lalgard, almost due south of Kathmandu on the Terai, the plains south of the mountains. Initially the surgery there was being provided by Dr Des Soares from Anandaban and Dr Richard

Schwarz from Pokhara. They took it in turns to fly in and stay for a week or two doing the required surgery. I went there in February 2002, to teach some surgery, and to do some lecturing, and then went on by car to Pokhara. This was a very new program, meeting a real need of the Nepalis from the plains, where leprosy was common, who could not easily go up to Kathmandu for their treatment.

Nepal of course, was a closed kingdom for many years. Once it became theoretically "open", in the early 1950s, the INF was granted permission to walk in from India and set up their first hospital in Pokhara, the original Shining Hospital. They built it using Quonset or Nissen huts – corrugated iron structures left over from World War 2 – and horribly hot in summer. To keep the heat down, the cleaners would shin up on ladders and literally scrub the corrugated iron roofs until they shone, making it marginally less hot inside. These shining huts could be seen for miles around, hence the "Shining Hospital". The Christians who ran it longed that it would also be a shining witness to the love of Jesus – and so it proved in that very needy country.

About the same time as INF was allowed in to set up that hospital, the UMN was given permission to set up the Patan Christian Hospital in Kathmandu. Originally, it occupied the ancestral mansion of one of the Nepali nobility, even having a stuffed deer head in the main hall! During the 1970s it was moved to one of the Durbas, official squares on the edge of Kathmandu, where it has expanded into quite a large, very well planned, well run facility, which includes a shoemaking and artificial limb factory. Patan was another centre that I worked in on several occasions.

In June, 2000, I was one of a group of specialists who met at Pokhara for a conference on The Management of the Neurologically Impaired/Neuropathic Lower Limb. There were about a dozen of us, each with our own specialty. We all presented papers, which were discussed, and the conclusions were published in the Leprosy Review. Later it formed the basis of a new textbook, *Surgical Reconstruction and Rehabilitation in Leprosy and other Neuropathies*, written by Richard Schwarz (surgeon) and Wim Brandsma (physiotherapist) – an excellent reference book.

Much of the medical work in Nepal has been done by volunteers, often, but not always, Christian missionaries. Societies like UMN and INF have provided medical personnel at no charge to the Nepalis. Another source of occasional help was the medicos who used to go for a week of mountain climbing and then might spend another week or two helping in one of the medical programs. Hundreds of Nepalis can thank them for lives saved, feet and hands reconstructed, and eyes treated to restore normal function.

When I first went into Nepal, the government seemed grateful for the help we gave, especially as they were not training any doctors of their own. In the last few years however Nepal, like many other countries, has decided that any medical personnel must formally register and pay an annual fee in order to work there. As a result many of the teams have stopped going. The size of the fee is not the problem so much as the time-consuming bureaucratic business – filling in papers and having to be interviewed by a committee. They may have prevented charlatans coming into Nepal as doctors – the supposed aim of the system – but they also deterred genuine willing and skilled volunteer workers.

Then came the appalling slaughter of the royal family, and the Maoist unrest became much more aggressive, making it much harder for visitors to stay and work in Nepal. The Leprosy Mission is still working at Anandaban but I have not been back there since February, 2003.

30

SYDNEY UNIVERSITY; AND "FUNNY FEET"

1977 proved a very busy year. It started with trips to India and Nepal, then Libya and back to Thailand. A few months later it was Hong Kong, Taiwan and Korea. Various letters had been chasing me around, regarding the recommendation that I should receive an Elected Fellowship of the Australasian College of Surgeons. After the presentation in October 1977, (see Chapter 27) I remained in Australia for deputation and a short leave.

During that stay I spent a couple of weeks at the Brisbane Medical School as Visiting Guest Lecturer, taking part in lectures, seminars and ward rounds, as well as taking TLM meetings. It was a busy and profitable three months, especially for the mission, and in sharing medical expertise with the teachers of the next generation.

Professor John Lowenthal, Professor of Surgery of Sydney University, invited me to take up a temporary lectureship in his Department. We decided that the most practical time would be 1979, when I was next due for home leave. In 1979 I came back from Asia by a different route. I flew into Perth, where I spoke at TLM meetings and taught at medical institutions. Then I took the Indian Pacific train – something I had dreamed of doing for many years – to Kalgoorlie, of gold rush fame, then to Adelaide so I could speak in both places about TLM work and also share some medical expertise.

In Adelaide I was asked to examine a few patients with leprosy and discuss their treatment. In every state of Australia there are leprosy patients if one knows where to look for them. A Chinese doctor, who had been in charge of the leprosy hospital at Singapore, had settled there and had become involved with leprosy patients, some of them migrants. Few local doctors would think of leprosy as a diagnosis. In Melbourne too, I spoke about the leprosy work to Mission supporters, and helped local doctors to diagnose and treat it and other conditions with which I was familiar, though my methods for management were different from those used in Australia. Then I came home to Sydney.

Here I was back with the family, and acquired a car for easy transport. The Warren home, now occupied by my brother Bill and his family, was my base. I worked at the University for three months from September to November 1979. There I met Garth Maxwell, who worked at the University and was very skilled with scientific and electrical equipment and gadgets. I was a speaker at a TLM seminar for medical personnel and anyone else that was interested. We asked Garth to be in charge of the technical equipment and I guess he became 'hooked'. He became a keen TLM supporter, and later joined the State Committee. For years he set up and ran many of our meetings and became a great encourager to me.

At about the time Garth was to retire from the university, he slipped and fell, cutting his right hand badly. The nerves were repaired by a surgeon who did a good job, but when it came to deciding how to restore function with all the severed tendons, the surgeon said: "I think you'd better wait till Grace comes back", as I was overseas at the time. We organised that I would do the operation with a particular hand surgeon at Royal North Shore Hospital. I did far more than I would usually do in one hand at one sitting. Professor Reeve came in to see what was happening and commented on how efficient I was in moving tendons around.

Garth was in a cast for about four weeks; then an experienced physiotherapist took over the job of re-educating his muscles, to give him back the functions that he needed. It was not 100 per cent restored – it is certainly not the best hand that I have reconstructed. The fact that all the nerves had been cut explains why it is so cold and does not sweat, and there are various other problems. But it works and is usable. Garth wears a mitten to keep it warm, but he is able to do everything he needs to. He can hold a screwdriver, and cords, lights and switches. Despite some difficulties, he can cope. He is even grateful that he has had a first-class experience of what it is like to have a hand reconstructed. When he is doing TLM deputation work, he does not hesitate to use his "show and tell" right hand to demonstrate that once it was useless and that now he is capable of doing a lot. It is wonderful how God brings people across our paths so that we are able to work together in God's service.

While I was at the university I was able to speak on neuropathy, leprosy and its surgery at the Monday morning meetings of the surgical professorial staff. I showed a slide of a young boy who had been born with an inability to feel pain. I had first met that boy, Sarli, then aged about 9, in the late 1960s in North Pakistan. I tell his story in chapters 10 and 21.

I pointed out that Sarli had a congenital neuropathy, not rare in Asian countries. One of the Australian surgeons said, "Oh, we do not see anything like that here." I did not respond; I did not need to. One of the other surgeons in the group said, "We certainly see it in South Africa." Little did I know, then, that in Australia within 20 years, I would be treating over 40 patients, all descendants of one migrant who arrived in 1800, with similar problems.

The congenital or familial abnormality of nerve function goes by several different names in medical textbooks, but is really the same basic problem. The patient starts off with some degree of abnormality that does not appear severe initially, but grows worse as he grows older. The problem is often only an inability to feel pain, but it can also result in muscle paralysis and even a complete inability to feel anything, and these people are then very prone to damage themselves just as in diabetes or leprosy. In congenital neuropathy the problem is not confined to feet; it may affect the hands and the feet equally, and it may slowly progress right up the limb until the whole limb has lost its ability to feel pain. It also has more problematic effects in some patients. So I was able to alert them to a problem that certainly did exist, but which was not common and is probably missed more often than it is recognised.

As part of the lectureship I was able to teach the medical students what I knew of neuropathy as it affected different diseases. I also had contacts with the Royal North Shore Hospital where Tom Taylor was Professor for Orthopaedics. His secretary offered to do some typing for me. This was before the computer revolution, and typing took a long time. Back then, she did the first typed version of the book that was eventually published in 1999!

One day on ward rounds in the university hospital, we saw a woman in bed with diabetes and ulcers on her feet. I had not done a lot with diabetes up to that point – I had treated a few patients in Asia, but in those days diabetes was not considered such a common disease in Asia as it was in Australia. (Now it **is** common in Asia and is virtually epidemic in Australia and other developed countries). The ulcers had developed because she did not feel pain normally – that is, her feet, as in leprosy, were neuropathic. She had been in and out of hospitals for eighteen months. On each admission, the ulcers seemed to improve but got worse as soon as she left hospital.

She was in hospital on bed rest, having all sorts of expensive but apparently ineffectual dressings put on her wounds: the traditional treatment for a diabetic ulcer in Australia. I know one thing: it is not the medication, the dressing or the antibiotics that heals the ulcer. I have been able to show that many ulcers will heal on adequate 'rest and protect' programs **without antibiotics**, but few will heal **on antibiotics without protection**. Though this woman was in hospital for bed rest, no one suggested that she should not walk at all! On this occasion the Professor, who was doing the rounds, suddenly turned to me and said: "Grace, you treat a lot of neuropathic ulcers; what would you do for this patient?" I gulped and said, "We would put her in a total contact cast, sir". "Righto, fair enough," he said, "Do it, and let's see what happens". So we did that. We allowed her to go home walking in the cast, returning once a week to have the ulcer checked. Lo and behold, within six weeks it was absolutely healed. In Hong Kong we had discovered that just one step a day on an ulcer is enough to destroy any healing that has occurred in the last 24 hours. By using that cast we achieved the essential rest and protection needed for healing.

So the total contact plaster cast was found to work to produce healing that had failed to occur previously, using the standard, accepted type of care. The second question was why she had developed such an ulcer in the first place. When making the cast, I noticed that her foot was abnormal in shape, although the X-ray had been reported as 'normal". I had my doubts! A radiologist did some further X-ray studies for me. We discovered that the patient had actually torn a tendon in her foot and there were fragments of bone still attached to that tendon. Small fractures that were not obvious in the initial X-rays could now, 18 months later, be identified. They had resulted in a deformity which was the basic reason for the ulcers. I pointed out the X-ray abnormality to the other surgeons – it was an uncorrected, unhealed fracture. To me it was not unusual but they had missed it completely. Once the ulcer was healed, we operated and repaired the torn tendon and reshaped the foot to reduce the chances of her getting further ulceration. She had to remain in a total contact walking cast for many months after that surgery. I had to hand over the case to another Sydney surgeon when I returned overseas, but I saw her later and found we had achieved a first class result. This was very gratifying, because she was one of the first non-leprosy patients I had responsibility for in Australia since receiving my surgical Fellowship. She stayed ulcer free until she died of other causes some years later.

I treated several other patients with good results and the staff soon realised that I knew what I was doing. We had some very interesting discussions on how you should do this casting and the variations that one could use. Others began to realise what could be done for patients with reduced pain perception in their feet. About this time I also treated a girl born with spina bifida, causing abnormal sensations in her feet and a degree of paralysis of her legs. She had chronic ulcers on both heels. It was a similar sort of thing: devising a cast so that there would be no pressure actually on the ulcers, so that the tissues could heal. Once again I was able to show that the ulcers in neuropathy will heal if they are protected from movement and trauma. Dr Paul Brand had realised, years before, that these casts that I use so frequently, increase the rate of healing.

One patient had a chronic ulcer on his foot due to a familial neuropathy that refused to heal. I put him in my usual cast and within three weeks the ulcer was healing and eventually healed extremely well. I wanted to operate on him early but it was not convenient. He got a friend to make him a special device so he could put the foot into a half splint and walk in that. So he was walking around in a split cast. At that time I was not using split casts – or modified removable total contact casts as they came to be known – but now I use them routinely for chronic foot problems. So that patient's inventiveness improved my methods of care! By the 1990s we had developed what we called the Bi-valved Modified Total Contact Cast. We have to use this long complicated name because people objected that it was not a true total contact cast. We use a little wool padding to allow dressings to be included and a liner to keep any dressings in place. Of course there must be co-operation; if the patient keeps taking the cast off and walking on the ulcer it will never heal.

These casts took on quite well, because specialists realised that here was an easy way of immobilising the foot so the patient could be treated at home without long hospital stays. Furthermore doctors or podiatrists could take the casts off easily and quickly in their rooms, do the dressings and re-apply them.

Another patient in the early 1990s was a man with a very severe form of diabetes, who had been in and out of hospital for years with ulcers on his feet. Once we had made a pair of these casts, for both feet at once, he could live at home. For the next ten years, he literally lived in his plaster casts. As one cast would wear out, we would make a new one, and although he did not live 'ulcer free', the ulcers he had were relatively superficial. So he could spend a lot more time at home, which suited him, and suited the hospital authorities also.

I've used the casts now very widely in Australia and I've taught people in other countries how to make them. It's been very challenging over the years, as I have been asked for advice and to help with the care of lots of patients with very problematic, complicated feet. One of my sayings is: "Don't say an ulcer won't heal until you have tried it for at least six weeks in a contact cast." All ulcers require rest and protection from trauma in order to heal. A foot that is in a total contact cast will heal much more quickly and much better than a foot that is left free, with the patient knocking and rubbing the ulcers, so destroying the body's attempts to heal itself even if the patient is not walking.

But I have raced ahead on my plaster cast hobby horse, beyond the story of that time at Sydney University and what followed. In that time I met lots of general, orthopaedic and other surgeons and also podiatrists looking after 'funny feet', and I was able to keep contact with many of them later on when I was working in Australia. But in those months in 1979 I gave them all something to think about. I have been very gratified to find that there are centres in Australia where the principles that I taught are still being applied today.

31

A String of Awards

I had returned to Asia and was getting on with my work when, about 1980, I learned that I'd been nominated as an elected Fellow of the Royal College of Surgeons, in London. Now this is the prestigious college – **THE** College – the original one. To receive an elected Fellowship to it there are a number of requirements. Somebody eligible has to nominate you; it was a long time before I ferreted out who had done so – a surgeon in Brisbane who had heard me lecturing there in 1977. I needed to receive the Fellowship in person, in London. When could I go to London? Other things intervened, but, early in 1984, I was able the make the trip and duly received the Fellowship – a great honour.

Later that year I was back in Sydney doing some work at the Sydney University medical school. One day I met Professor Tom Reeve in the corridor; "Oh Grace" he said, "have you got a list of your publications?" I said, "Well, not with me". "Can you get it for me, in a hurry?" The Tropical Medicine School on request produced a nice long list of the articles that I had written, all correctly coded. I was able to rustle up my CV and to get it all to him the next day when he wanted it. He just wanted it in a hurry – I did not know the reason. I found out later that, as Dean of the Faculty of Medicine, he was on the committee organizing the big ceremony to be held in 1985 for the centenary of the first women to graduate. He was looking for female medical graduates deemed to merit an honorary doctorate. Well, I had my Master of Surgery which was academically equivalent to a doctorate, and I was a graduate of Sydney University. So Professor Reeve kindly put me up for an MD, Honoris Causa.

I spent the first part of 1985 in Asia. But I needed to return to

Sydney to collect this honorary MD. As a missionary I could not afford an extra trip from Bangkok to Sydney, nor could I expect TLM to fund it – it was not work. But a letter came from church friends with a cheque to cover the air fare. The Lord knows my needs and often meets them before I ask! So there I was on the big night in May 1985. Five women were receiving honorary doctorates: two in medicine, one in law, and two in arts. That was a big thrill – and another degree to go after my name.

I headed off overseas again and buzzed around Asia teaching here and there. In November 1985, I was in Hong Kong, staying in the YMCA. A royal event was on, and I was sitting up enjoying the TV pageantry when the phone rang. It was Australia calling. A government official wanted to know if I would be prepared to accept the award of Member of the Order of Australia, to be given in the Australia Day honours list in 1986. I have never found out who nominated me for that, though I have my ideas. I could not be home in Australia at the time the 1986 Australia Day honours list was published, but I was able to go later in the year to receive the award from the Governor of New South Wales. Fascinating, is not it! Here's this girl who could barely get through her medical course – what is God doing for her? Well!

Later, in 1986, I was talking to some of my English colleagues when one of them suggested, "Why do not you apply for a Hunterian lectureship? This work that you're doing with neuropathic feet is not well recorded. Most people do not know how to treat ulcers. It would make an excellent paper." He suggested I call it *The Conservative Management of the Neuropathic Foot* – in contradistinction to pure surgery. This was because, as far as possible, I did not operate on these feet, but tried to treat them in a conservative way. So I prepared a rough draft and submitted the necessary précis. I was duly awarded a professorship of the Royal College of Surgeons of England for the year 1986/87 and had to go there to read the lecture to the College early in 1987. That was a thrilling night for me. There I was, lecturing the professors! I gave my lecture, about forty-five minutes in length, and before presenting me with a commemorative medal, the Professor, who was chairing the meeting said, "Thank you very much, Dr Warren. You've brought us back to the first principles that we have all forgotten. Most of us are getting so sophisticated that we forget that the basic needs of a damaged foot are rest and protection." So in the space of those few years in the eighties I added to my trophies an Order of Australia, the Fellowship of the Royal College of Surgeons, and the Hunterian Lectureship Medal.

Academic recognition is one thing, but in many ways I value more the many opportunities I have had to influence people in other ways. I collect quotations and sayings, and one of them is: "If you want to send an idea around the world, wrap it in a man or a woman." In contrast to that, there is no way a man or a woman can go everywhere, so if you want to get an idea around the world you also need to get it into print. What's more you have got to get it into print in a book or a magazine which is reliable and highly regarded, so that people will believe what you say and act on it. So throughout the 1980s and 1990s I continued to write articles for reputable medical journals. When Professor Reeve asked for my list of publications I guess there were thirty. There are a lot more now.

In 1984 I was asked to do a couple of chapters on leprosy and leprosy surgery for a text called *Surgery for All*, edited by Timothy Harrison who was working at the Aga Khan Medical School in Karachi. Professor Bruce Conolly asked me at one stage, for illustrations for a book on hand lesions and deformities. It is full of the most beautiful coloured pictures (well, I think they are beautiful!) of different conditions of hands, with instructions as to how they should be treated. So some of my many clinical pictures were being used in a wider field. Then, in the 1990s, Bruce asked me if I could write chapters for a book which he called *Atlas of Hand Surgery*, a "How to ..." production full of detailed line drawings. It took me quite a while to produce those chapters, which included procedures I did not normally do, working together with Bruce. I ended up with four chapters in that book. When somebody asks "How do you do so and so?" it is marvellous to be able to go and get Professor Conolly's book. It's all there in detail, enough to enable even a surgeon new to the procedure to get a good result. The diagrams were line drawings done by a highly qualified illustrator whom I got to know reasonably well – Levant Efe. He had graduated in medicine in Turkey, and from there, went to North America where he studied medical illustration. Then he moved to Australia and now works in Melbourne. Besides doing beautiful diagrams he has highly developed skills in computer graphics. In my chapters some of the diagrams are ones I did myself – probably touched up by the artist, but nevertheless still my drawings.

There was another surgical textbook covering basically the surgery of leprosy, in which I have a couple of chapters, and there are other textbooks for which I've done sections or part chapters. More and more people are realising that the simple techniques, which are effective, have basically been forgotten in today's flood of high tech medicine and surgery. Over the years, whenever I've come to Australia, I've been asked to see, give advice and to operate on a certain number of patients who have deformities of the hand. Professor Conolly was one who recognised fairly early that I'd had to deal with all sorts of hand deformities, not just the routine ones of leprosy. So he would often invite me to a clinic to join in discussions about complicated hands. Quite frequently I've been asked to prepare papers and speak to medical conferences or to take part in discussion groups. Once I officially retired, I could attend most of the major scientific meetings of the Australasian College of Surgeons and present papers.

As well as the papers presented at conferences there are poster displays. You can prepare them all beforehand. On registering you get your site for displays and put up your posters, which stay up all week, so people can study them again and again. I developed the habit of turning up at these conferences with several – I think my maximum was ten – different sets of these teaching posters. I'd hang around between sessions to talk to people and answer questions about what can be done for people with neuropathy. So I have been spreading the word more and more widely – how effectively I may never know. But if some people are saved from losing limbs surely that is worthwhile!

My life has certainly never been restricted. When I am in medical circles and they hear that I do faces, hands and feet some people raise their eyebrows in horror. I remember an orthopaedic conference in Singapore back in 1966 where I met Ken Clezy for the first time. In medical matters we immediately bonded. One day we were talking to another person, who did leprosy surgery, and spoke about nose reconstructions. One of the orthopaedic surgeons came along and said: "Nose reconstructions? This is an orthopaedic conference!" This was on the pedantic grounds that cartilage, not bone, forms the shape of the nose. Ken turned to him and said: "Yes, I know it is, but we do use the iliac crest (i.e. the hip bone) to reconstruct the nose, and that is orthopaedic, is not it?" He did not know what to say to that! I guess that mirrors a lot of what we do, because a leprosy rehabilitation surgeon will cross boundaries to do all that is possible to help a patient.

One of the problems of leprosy is a paralysis of the facial muscles. Fortunately, this usually only affects one side of the face and it is usually only the upper half of the face. The problem may be one of being unable to shut one eye properly, causing it to leak tears a lot with a staring, wide-open look. The patient is likely to get all sorts of infections in the eye with dust and dirt and other problems that may result in blindness. Now, by reconstructive surgery, we bring another muscle in from the side of the head and use that to make the eyelid shut. It's a fascinating thing to do. It's technically not difficult and yet it must be done perfectly or it won't work.

There is a nice story of a patient who had had a muscle transfer so that he could close his eyelids. The muscle that we use is one used for chewing. Dining in a restaurant one night he was shocked when the waitress suddenly slapped his face. "Oh," she said, "You keep winking at me!" Poor guy! Every time he chewed his meat he winked – apparently at the waitress! Making patients wink at the girls is a small price to pay in order to save their vision and make them look more normal most of the time!

This was a procedure that I learnt in the 1960s. I worked out my own modification of it and have done it dozens of times since. I remember one session with a general surgeon doing it in Singapore for a young school teacher, who had had encephalitis as a child and was left with a deformity of the face. The surgeon had asked if I could do anything to help. If I would do the operation he was more than happy to have her on his own list and that he would assist me. When we'd finished, he said he'd never seen it done before. He was fascinated. I do not think he had even heard of it. He said "Well, Dr Warren, that is very interesting. Do you do many of those?" With a mischievous grin I said: "Well, last month in Pakistan we did thirteen". That's typical of the number of patients that we get in leprosy. If a surgeon like him had done thirteen in his lifetime he would think his experience was extensive. Once, in Australia I was about to operate on a youth of 17 with foot problems due to spina bifida. He said, "I do not want to be used as a guinea pig, Dr Warren – how many of these operations have you done?" "Oh, at least a thousand," I assured him. After that he let me go ahead!

People at home were trying to tap this vast experience. In 1990 I was asked to write an editorial on facial surgery which was published by the Australian and New Zealand Journal of Ophthalmology. As a result I've had a number of requests for details of how to do some of these procedures. Some say I am old-fashioned in doing that particular muscle transplant for this type of facial paralysis. But it works and it works quickly. Within six weeks of the surgery the patient should be looking basically normal and be able to shut the eye at will. How much physiotherapy the patient does affects how well the reconstructed, reactivated face works and appears.

Thinking back on this period in the eighties when so many awards and honours came my way, I am still amazed and humbled. Missionaries are not generally admired in a hard-headed secular world. However, if they are clearly into "good works", especially in the medical line, they are more likely to meet respect or at least a grudging approval. Some may have thought that, by going off to serve abroad, I had thrown away my chances of normal medical advancement and "sacrificed" a comfortable and successful life as a doctor here. I suppose I would have become a GP. But Christians have a saying, "God is no man's debtor". In my case, because I followed his leading and worked with leprosy patients, among the most miserably despised and needy people in undeveloped countries, God eventually made possible the winning of high academic and professional recognition. I suppose it just goes to show that God loves to reverse the world's values.

32

The '80s – The World my Theatre

By the end of the 1970s I had established a pattern of work which was taking me regularly to a large number of centres in about ten Asian countries, some once a year, some more often, usually for two to three weeks in each place at one time, teaching and treating patients to improve the long term quality of leprosy care. Some were Leprosy Mission hospitals, while the others were run by a very wide range of groups and organizations.

It was fascinating to see how groups generally were willing to set aside their own social, religious and medical prejudices and accept me, a woman, doing leprosy work as a Christian service. Well, I was prepared to come to them, to work with them, seeing their patients and helping them to deal with their own problems. Moreover, I was training them to carry on the work when I had gone. They knew I was part of TLM International, and it was often possible for the mission to provide reference books or equipment if needed. This was more practical than sending their doctors away, to places where, although they would receive good training, they would not always learn what was needed for their institution. The various countries have very different principles and practice in leprosy work. Each racial group has its own variation on how leprosy presents and how it should be treated, and, unless we are prepared to adapt to those variations, we may not meet the need of those particular patients. An example: in the sixties I visited a Korean institution after the doctors had studied in India. There were terrible foot problems. I asked them, "Weren't you taught what sort of shoes to provide for your patients? "Oh, yes," they said, "they told us to provide sandals, but how can you put a patient into sandals when it is snowing?" Good question! All principles of care need adapting to local conditions, and because they had not been taught principles or application, they failed to seek the right type of footwear for patients in Korea's cold climate.

But now the local workers were finding that here was a doctor prepared to come to their hospital and help; to help them adapt to the various situations and to deal with their problems using equipment locally available; a doctor sponsored by TLM at no cost to them.

In the 1980s I was on a regular run going round these institutions, examining, teaching procedures, training nurses, physiotherapists and others, so that they would be able to carry on with the work. I guess some might sneer, "Jack of all trades and master of none!" Maybe so, but thanks to God's goodness and to his giving me the right people in the right place at the right time, I was "Jill of all trades and master of one." I had a Master of Surgery degree, followed by a Fellowship of the Royal College of Surgeons. This meant that the third world countries that were becoming very degree conscious, were quite satisfied with my card with four or five degrees listed after my name. I was obviously "well studied" as one lecture chairman put it while introducing me. Little did he realise how I'd got those letters after my name – not by academic study at all, but by hands-on practical work in the field – but it satisfied him and his colleagues that I knew what I was doing. It was God who got me those degrees. He knew they would make me academically acceptable – though not a better surgeon or teacher.

Pakistan: Here I had the approval of the government and was welcomed by them. Originally I worked in the government leprosarium, but then later I made my headquarters in the non-government Marie Adelaide Leprosy Centre, because that was the major training centre for the paramedicals who were working right across the country in the government institutions. I visited Pakistan approximately every second year and have dealt with that in detail in Chapter 22.

Bangladesh: I went in with the Christian missions, but I was soon accepted and welcomed by the government authorities. Every time I went there, I had to go and have an interview with the government head of the leprosy division to discuss their program.

Virtually every year I routinely visited various hospitals. It was gratifying to see the programs develop and the leadership often taken over by the local doctors. A main centre was the British Baptist Mission centre at Chandraghona, right down in the south eastern corner in the Chittagong hill tracts. This is one of the less controlled areas where there are many tribal people. The British Baptist hospital – a very good one – for many years included a leprosy centre. An English surgeon, Bob Hart, worked there and was doing some reconstructive surgery. We operated on a number of patients together. One patient there featured in Christian literature in the 1980s. Her severely affected legs and feet had required amputation. On two artificial legs, she was a good example of what modern medicine, surgery and prosthetics can do to enable the disabled to continue to live at home and look after themselves and their families.

Nepal: I went into Nepal as a tourist in 1973. Then in 1976 and 1978 I went to help at Anandaban TLM Hospital. In 1979 I started to go in and out helping in the training programs, in both Pokhara and Anandaban, teaching, consulting, lecturing, and assisting. Those two programs have continued and have done really well. Both also take patients with deformities that are not due to leprosy.

The one at Pokhara is connected with the local government general hospital and there is now also a medical college there. Medical students, who might otherwise be clueless, are sent down to the leprosy hospital to learn something about leprosy. We also taught some of the government doctors the essentials, training them in the basics of how to recognise and diagnose leprosy and treat it. They could do this for the patients who were coming and going in the regular clinics and centres where these doctors worked. Thus the work in Nepal got onto a very good footing.

India: Often in the eighties I was visiting clinics in India, a country with enormous numbers of leprosy patients. Back in the 70s, the government acknowledged that there were probably four million people in India with leprosy. That included people who had completed treatment and people who were still receiving it.

One highlight in 1980 was an excellent conference at Karigiri at which my friend and mentor, Paul Brand, was one of the main speakers, discussing the problems of loss of nerve function and its consequences. Methods of measuring function and management were discussed and trials were worked out for testing different methods. People from many countries and backgrounds participated in that conference, and now more than twenty years later, it is clear that we have certainly made many advances in the understanding and management of leprosy and neuropathic problems.

Thailand: In 1980 my base was still Manorom Christian Hospital in Central Thailand. I was going up to Chiang Mai about every three months to do the surgery at the McKean Rehabilitation Institute, owned by the Church of Christ of Thailand, at which Trevor Smith from TLM Australia was the doctor in charge. Trevor did the routine surgery. Anything that was unusual he preferred to hand over to somebody with more experience. He too was admitting a good number of people with disabilities from other causes. McKean underwent a complete transformation and a beautiful new rehabilitation unit was built, with a big, well-equipped room for the physiotherapy and occupational therapy. The excellent prosthetics workshop was presided over by Mr Teng, whom I had first met at Manorom in 1962 where he was a leprosy patient and shoemaker. We had done some work on his hands and feet to reduce his disability, and he worked in Chiang Mai for the rest of his days, making shoes with various types of orthotics for the leprosy patients.

In 1982 the Mission held an international conference in Chiang Mai. As a result I was asked if I could go to the refugee camps on the Thai-Cambodia border to assist in the care of leprosy patients. I was warned that I would be merely instructing and would not be able to do any surgery, because the Red Cross provided all surgery in the camps, and for obvious reasons, it was basically restricted to emergency cases.

I arrived at the camp early one morning to be greeted with a message that the Red Cross unit had an Australian team in charge that quarter. The leader of the team had asked if I could go to his office on arrival. I was delighted to discover it was Dr James Ellis, who, only a couple of months earlier in Australia, had organised treatment for some arthritis in my back! Jim knew what I could do; he had operated with me in Australia, so he set me straight to work operating on a refugee patient. He described the patient as a "psychological emergency". He had attempted suicide a few weeks earlier because he could see no future in life due to the deformities of his hands.

Jim also negotiated with the Red Cross so that later, whenever I went in to the camp, I was politely asked: "When would you like the operating room?" I probably did 10-20 operations each time I visited. I went there every 2-3 months from mid-1982 to the early 1990s, about the time the camps closed. We were able to teach the workers how to help many of the patients by physiotherapy and self care, and succeeded in improving function and/or appearance for dozens of leprosy patients and others with similar disabilities. Finding Jim Ellis there and the open door he provided for me to work in the camps was just another of those "God-incidences", those special happenings that God organises to help those in need.

Medical students frequently came to do their electives with us. In the early eighties, Scott Murray came and assisted me. Later he returned as the surgeon for Manorom Hospital and also worked at McKean.

There was also the OMF hospital in Saiburi, South Thailand. Here, as in many other parts of the world, the government provided a leprosy service, coming in to examine patients and do surveys. They would provide six or twelve months of medical treatment for leprosy patients, but there was no one there for the rest of the time to deal with their complications and problems, and certainly no physiotherapist or shoemaker. The patients soon discovered that, although they got their medicines free from the government – a fact which suited us because they were expensive – they would come to us for management of their complications. So these patients were being looked after by both groups. Here was another example of good cooperation between Christian missions and the government.

In Thailand I regularly visited the government hospital at Phrapradaeng where the senior surgeon was Dr Ake (see Chapter 24) who was involved in my being asked to lecture on leprosy at the Government International Dermatology course held annually in Bangkok. Of course my teaching slides were international – including all skin colours and many countries. As the students were from all over Asia, that was important. I enjoyed meeting some of those students elsewhere in Asia when I went to help with local programs.

In the mid-eighties I was asked to take part in a government survey in the Uthai area just west of Manorom. The other consultant was a Japanese leprosy specialist who was very good to work with. We examined literally dozens of Thai people who lived in the area. One woman was very interesting. The paramedical workers had brought her in, suspecting leprosy. She had two anaesthetic patches, one on her leg just above the left knee and another just below the left elbow. We carefully checked her all over and could find nothing else suggestive of leprosy. Then we got one of the Thai interpreters in to help us. After all we were two foreigners.

The solution was fascinating. She was about 50 years of age, and, as a typical rural Thai woman, she had from an early age been involved in planting rice. To do that the women wade in the muddy water and hold a handful of rice seedlings in their left hand. The elbow of the left arm rests on the thigh just above the knee while the worker bends over to plant a seedling deep in the mud and water. She had spent many hours every day in this position for many years, with her weight supported in part by her elbow pressing on the leg above the bent knee. The constant pressure had resulted in the death of the nerves in the contact areas, and these were the darkish spots which had lost their feeling! An easy answer once you worked it out. It is a perfect example of how one really needs to know local customs if one's medical and diagnostic work is to be effective.

Hong Kong: I still continued to make the occasional visit to Hong Kong, seeing any new patients. Dr Norman Honey from the UK was the doctor in charge after I left Hong Kong and he managed the leprosy clinics very well for a number of years. I discussed things with him and also with one or two of the surgeons who were prepared to operate on the leprosy patients.

The patients in Hong Kong were relatively well cared for. Those who needed hospitalisation were accommodated in Lai Chi Kok Hospital. If surgery was needed they were just admitted to an ordinary orthopaedic unit in a government hospital. The persistent and lingering Chinese fear of the disease meant that the leprosy patients were never treated quite the same as everybody else, but, aided by social welfare, they were able to live in the big resettlement blocks, and many managed to get government jobs. So they were really quite well off compared with a lot of other leprosy patients that I have treated around Asia.

Taiwan: From Hong Kong I also continued to go to Taiwan. I was doing clinics in Taiwan for the best part of twenty years. Again there were interesting problems. For instance, one patient turned up at a clinic with a note from the local medical school to say that she had leprosy. Would we please take her? I did not think she had leprosy at all. We carefully took her history. She had some lesions and the fingers of her right hand were clawed, just like a typical leprosy hand. However, we learned that the damaged hand had been the result of a car accident many years before. It was completely unrelated to the lesions, which were due to tuberculosis.

South Korea: I visited Korea less often in the 1980s. The old leprosy colonies that were so well populated in the 1950s and 1960s, with segregation compulsory under Japanese occupation, had now become regular villages with many non-leprosy patients living in them. I enjoyed visits down south to the Il Sin Hospital in Pusan, as some of the staff I knew were still working there. Visits to Korea were almost a holiday compared with the pressure of work in other Asian centres.

In 1982 I was invited by the Australasian College of Surgeons to address the Tasmanian members at their annual scientific meeting. In order to do that I took my car across on the Bass Strait ferry and combined the conference with other medical work and with TLM deputation. Kathleen Collett came down to join me in Hobart and we did some touring and sightseeing. It was fascinating to find out how much I remembered of the days when I had lived in Cullenswood as a young child in 1933/34.

I visited **Africa** again in 1988 and started the regular trips to **Israel**. Both of these feature in their own chapters, and arose out of my trip to Europe for the International Leprosy Association International congress at The Hague in Holland in 1988, which was again an excellent chance to meet and confer with colleagues from around the world, and to seek to spread my work and methods of saving neuropathic limbs. It was always good at these Conferences to be able to talk to Paul Brand and Stanley Browne, and others who were the leaders in updating leprosy care in general.

That was the last of those conferences for me. After it I was able to spend time in England with Dr Michael Waters at the School of

Tropical Medicine in London, where I also did some surgery.

My diary for the eighties reads like a travelogue, backwards and forwards across Asia and visiting many other places as well. Work in Singapore and Malaysia slackened off after 1975, and, by the eighties, became rare and visits were usually of short duration. In retrospect I realised that, in the fifteen years between 1975 and 1989, as I was running "in-service" training courses in ten Asian countries, I did not spend more than three weeks in any one place at any one time – even when I was on so-called "leave" in Australia.

It never ceases to amaze me that, in spite of the hundreds of journeys and millions of kilometres I have flown in the course of my career, I was never involved in a real mishap, and only occasionally did I even experience significant flight delays. I praise God that He most certainly had his hand in the organisation of my many schedules, fitting things in and booking travel plans!

33

In and out of Israel

I first visited Israel in 1973, purely as a tourist. Kathleen Collett and I were on our way to the Leprosy Congress at Bergen in Norway. I had "done" Israel and was not hankering to go back. But a letter came from TLM early in 1988 to ask if it was possible for me to do some reconstructive surgery in Israel.

Israel had a small leprosy program, and Jean Gardiner, a physiotherapist originally from Sydney, was working there. She had worked with TLM and spent years in Hong Kong, Taiwan, Thailand and Indonesia. When she retired she volunteered to go to Israel and do some physiotherapy for the leprosy program there.

Jean worked at the Hansen Hospital in Jerusalem, where there were about 60 resident patients and maybe as many more outpatients. She realized that there were a number of people with deformities and that no-one was offering them any kind of reconstructive surgery, although some had been done in earlier decades. She had written to TLM asking if somebody could come and help – and the mission had decided that I was that somebody.

So it was that, in conjunction with my trip to The Hague in Holland for the Leprosy Congress of 1988, I was scheduled to go to Israel to do reconstructive surgery. I started off on a bad foot, as a flight mix-up meant I had to find my own way to Jerusalem from Tel Aviv. I arrived eventually at the Hansen Leprosy Hospital with Jean's list of patients, but it was hardly an ideal way to commence a program.

That was a relatively short trip. I did five operations and lectured on leprosy at a number of centres, including the Hansen Hospital itself, to the delight of the doctor in charge of the program. He greatly appreciated having somebody with an international reputation visiting his hospital to lecture and teach on his specialty of leprosy. This brought him recognition for what was a very much neglected specialty in the medical program in Israel at that time.

He invited me to come back to Israel whenever I liked to teach, lecture and treat patients. So over the next ten to fifteen years I went back to Israel almost every year, usually in the pleasantest seasons, spring and autumn, when I lectured in various colleges and hospitals and taught clinicians. I would see patients with complications and discuss difficult cases, advising on different forms of treatment, both medical and surgical, but I rarely did any surgery after that first visit.

Back then, I was very surprised to find that they had just over 300 patients on their cumulative register. But many, perhaps even more than 50%, had not been seen for years. If patients wanted more dapsone, the drug they used most for leprosy, they just wrote in and asked for it. It was sent to them and no one was monitoring their progress. If a patient developed a lepra reaction or an acute neuritis there was nowhere else to go except to the Hansen Leprosy Hospital in Jerusalem.

By 1988 the leprosy world had become very aware of the problems of dapsone resistance, of the dangers of giving dapsone as monotherapy – that is, making it the only drug in the treatment of active leprosy – and also of the dangers of giving it in a low dose. Israeli patients were definitely getting low doses. With medicines just posted to the patient, there was no way of checking on compliance. Did the patient take the medicine every day, or three times a week, as instructed? With no checks and no adequate charts to show their clinical progress, there was no record of whether or not they were suffering increasing levels of nerve damage, such as a loss of sensation, or whether they were developing paralysis of hands or feet or face. Although in theory this group of patients in

Israel were on treatment, in reality many were not being treated at all adequately.

I took upon myself the task of trying to teach the staff how leprosy ought to be treated in the world of 1988, with good record-keeping, and due respect to the fact that the problem of dapsone resistance was very much present in many of the countries that these patients came from.

Israel was at that time in the midst of a big program of encouraging Jewish communities in other countries, including third world countries, to make *aliyah* – to come and make Israel their home. It was a most unusual situation. Many of the immigrants came from countries with endemic leprosy, where leprosy had been treated for years. There was a big group of Ethiopian migrants, and I knew of a lot of dapsone resistance in Ethiopia. Fortunately, Dr Campbell Miller was seconded from the International Christian Embassy to help at the Hansen Hospital, and he supervised their treatment. He had treated leprosy in Ethiopia and spoke Amharic, their main language.

There were also Jews from India, Yemen, Lebanon and other areas where leprosy is endemic. In treating these people one needed to be aware of the fact that they might have arrived with dapsone resistance already. Unless they received another drug as well as dapsone, their disease could get worse.

I was able to show the staff some simple testing techniques and how to distinguish between a lepra reaction and a true relapse. I recommended the full multi-drug therapy (MDT), which was not being given at all in Israel at that time. Well, my suggestion to introduce MDT exploded like a bombshell! I was told very sternly that "No, we do ***not*** use MDT. It is not necessary." However a month or so after I left, the nurse, Ruthie, who was then in charge of the hospital, wrote to tell me that MDT **was** being used. So the staff did learn, even if they were not prepared to let me know it!

Ruth Wexler was a young Israeli woman, already a fully trained and experienced nurse, who, in 1988 had been appointed as the head nurse of the hospital to replace a man who had held the position for many years. She had been there only about two months when I arrived, and was only too glad to learn anything she could of leprosy. As it was obvious that this was going to be her job for the next ten years or so, I arranged with TLM International that Ruthie should go to Thailand, where she could work with me at Manorom Hospital for a week or two, and then go up to Chiang Mai to work with Trevor Smith at McKean for a month. This would give her a maximum chance of seeing patients with different forms of leprosy and with various complications. She would work with those being treated for ulcers, for reactions and having reconstructive surgery.

Was that providential – God's timing – or merely a matter of chance? In her very responsible new job, it was so vital for her to have adequate training, and the fact that I came just at that time meant she could receive it. Otherwise the treatment of leprosy in Israel would have continued to be far less than satisfactory. Ruthie came to Thailand in January, 1989. She was only able to spend four weeks instead of the six weeks originally planned, but she was an extremely capable student and learnt a lot about leprosy work in that time.

So in Israel, after 1989, I had a head nurse who was very intelligent, very capable and very interested in the patients' general welfare. If a patient came in with a real problem she would send me a note or a phone message, and I would ring her up and we'd have a long discussion on the phone. I would tell her what the patient needed and she would tell the doctor what I had said – and usually it would be done.

Now thanks to her efforts, all the patients on the cumulative list have been checked. It was found that some were listed two or three times, or had two identity cards. Some thought double doses of drugs would cure them more quickly. It was also found that a number did not have leprosy at all.

So by the early 2000s there were only about 240 patients on the list, and they were all being checked at least once a year, for any sign of active disease or treatment for complications or other conditions. All the patients, who had only been on low dosage dapsone as monotherapy for years, were given the WHO-recommended two years' treatment with MDT, so that their chances of relapsing would be reduced to a minimum.

Thus in the years between 1988 and 2002, the changes in the leprosy situation in Israel were tremendous, with the result that there are now far fewer problems and complications. Once Ruthie had seen what could be done, we were able to concentrate on the problems of foot care, foot ulcers and footwear.

Jean Gardiner had worked there in about 1987-89 as a volunteer physiotherapist. She was in Jerusalem for my first one or two visits, but illness then forced her to return home to Australia. She died a couple of years later from cancer. This meant that there was not anyone doing adequate physiotherapy, except what Ruthie could do from what she had learnt in Thailand. Well, one nurse cannot do everything, not when there were still twenty or so patients resident in the hospital!

An Israeli therapist, Hanna Melchior, was appointed to work with Ruthie. Hanna did the physio and foot care and taught the patients how to care for themselves. But initially she did not know much about leprosy. So TLM arranged for Chrissie Hoskins, an occupational therapist/hand therapist from UK, to come out to Israel to work with Hanna, teaching her to do testing of hands, testing of muscle power and sensation, and teaching the exercises that would help maintain hands, feet and faces in a socially acceptable way. Over the years Hanna became a real expert and she and Ruthie formed a fine, well recognized team.

Chrissie remained in Jerusalem for a couple of years. I did not see much of her because she was also doing work in the West Bank, where she had good associations with a Palestinian physiotherapist, Osama. In those days we were able to go in and out of Israel and the occupied territories without too much trouble. Osama was a tutor in the Palestinian physiotherapy school, and on one or two occasions he asked me to go in and lecture on hand and foot care in neuropathy.

In the early 90s I went into the West Bank on a number of occasions, mainly to lecture doctors and physiotherapists. One year there was a curfew, so it was difficult for a Westerner to go through the checkpoint into Ramallah. Chrissie and I needed to go, so we dressed appropriately in Palestinian-type clothes and head scarves and walked to the Arab taxi stand beside the Damascus Gate of the Old City of Jerusalem. There we got into an Arab taxi, Chrissie gave orders in Arabic and off we went. No trouble getting in, or getting back!

Osama introduced us to an Arab taxi driver who could work in Israel, and thereafter, if I needed to go to Ramallah, I would walk through the checkpoint in Bethlehem – no trouble – and meet by prior arrangement my friendly taxi driver who would take me the long way round to Ramallah. He would also pick me up in Jerusalem and take me to Gaza on some of my trips there to lecture and see patients. In these territories they never managed to set up a reliable clinic, and Palestinian patients came to Jerusalem for treatment. This meant that there was no follow up of contacts to see if there was leprosy in the family.

It is a joy now in the 21st century to see the old Hansen Hospital in Jerusalem still functioning, although only as an outpatients facility. It's a beautiful old building, built in the 1880s by Moravian missionaries. The walls are in some places a metre thick, solid blocks of stone, beautifully cool in summer – but like an ice-block in winter.

In Israel, now patients rarely need hospitalization for their leprosy. Most of them come in from all over Israel just for the day to be seen and then go home again. If they have other medical conditions that need to be treated, this is done by their own medical services. Ruthie keeps in constant touch with the family physician or medical service. She explains the needs of the leprosy patient and helps to coordinate any other medication that is needed so that the patients will continue to do well. She and Hannah also teach physiotherapy and arrange suitable footwear.

On those visits to Israel from 1988 to 2003 I had discussions with various surgeons on leprosy problems and the management of other similar medical conditions. I would often lecture on these subjects. A couple of the surgeons were quite keen to learn what was needed and would themselves do the procedure for the patient after I had gone. Occasionally I would recommend what I knew was appropriate for the patient's disability, but the local surgeon would decide that he knew better and would try something else. One or two of those surgical attempts failed to achieve the desired result and the patients were far from happy with the outcome. For that I was sorry, but one can only try to teach what will work.

Going into Israel each year for those 13 trips, my aim was to get the program running better and more smoothly. I think, on the whole, that was achieved. The most important object was to encourage both the local staff and the patients themselves to do what they could and should do, in the best interests of the patients. The result we wanted to see was that there would be a best practice situation for dealing with leprosy in Israel.

At times we had fascinating patients. In Israel there are patients who have immigrated, already obviously affected by leprosy. A few have caught leprosy while in Israel, but usually the patient has arrived as an immigrant without obvious signs of leprosy, and these appear a few years later. These signs are often misdiagnosed, because of the fact that if you do not think about leprosy you will never diagnose it.

When I am lecturing medical students I try to encourage them to put the possibility of leprosy on their differential diagnosis list so that they will at least think of it as a possibility. Then they can rule it out – but **not** without considering it. I will even say that, in a person who has ever visited or lived in an endemic leprosy country, any non-irritant skin lesion which has been present for more than six weeks should be considered as leprosy, until some other definite diagnosis has been made or until leprosy has been ruled out. Ruling out leprosy may not be easy, because unless the doctor actually asks "Is this leprosy?" it will probably not be considered as a possibility. Many pathologists are in that position. Examining a slide or specimen from a patient, they will never consider leprosy as the possible diagnosis because it is just too rare. "We never see leprosy in this country", they say. Yet for many of the forms of leprosy, a biopsy is the only way of being sure of the correct diagnosis.

A classic example of this occurred in Israel in the 1990s. There was an influx of refugees from Ethiopia – whole planeloads of them on charter flights and they were all meant to be checked for leprosy. Obviously some of them had been treated and the disease appeared quiescent; many were not diagnosed as having leprosy. Some of them could have been incubating the disease and it was not picked up. But a number of them were referred straight to us soon after they arrived for us to confirm diagnosis and to start treatment.

One day I saw a relatively young woman. A local doctor had treated her for a patch on her arm but it did not seem to heal up with cortisone cream. So he sent her to us for diagnosis. One of the first rules in leprosy is to examine the whole patient – and I mean the **whole** patient. Ideally, all clothes must be off. Social rules in some countries will not permit this, so you have to check all the skin little by little, but you can still achieve it. I found a suspicious anaesthetic lesion high up on this woman's thigh. She was not worried about it. I took a biopsy which we then sent up to the Haddassah Hospital to the pathology department. In due course – by this time I was back in Sydney – Ruthie informed me that the report said there was no evidence of leprosy. I said, "Sorry, that is crazy! There was no nerve function in that area. Did he describe the nerves that he could see in the biopsy?"

There had been no comment about nerves, so I said to Ruthie, "Please ask the pathologist to send me some slides, so I can have a look at them myself." In due course a box of four glass slides arrived. At the Royal North Shore Hospital I introduced myself to the pathology professor and explained to her that I had some slides taken from a patient overseas that I was convinced had leprosy. "I would very much like to look at them."

"Oh yes" she said, "by all means, and I've got a nice binocular microscope. May I have a look with you? I'd love to see a leprosy slide." I gave her the slides to set up. Almost at once she identified that it showed leprosy pathology.

After that, with any doubtful cases we used to send our biopsy slides off to England for diagnosis. If we had enough tissue we sent it to the local people as well, because I wanted to teach them how to do it. An incorrect diagnosis is sad, especially when we have gone to the trouble of taking a biopsy from the patient.

Whenever I visited Israel I was based in Jerusalem, but we were constantly travelling to other centres to see the local practitioners caring for patients, and to visit the medical schools. In the 1990s I was usually driven by Dr Campbell Miller of the International Christian Embassy. They had donated an ambulance for the leprosy program. After about 2000 with the *intifada,* the security situation became more risky. I was advised never to use public transport, even for short trips within Jerusalem. Ruthie took over the driving to outlying clinics in a private car and I used taxis, not buses, when in

Jerusalem. At that time I was staying with Jim and Maxine Carlill, fellow Australians living in Jerusalem helping with the work of the International Christian Embassy.

In 2003 we lectured at the medical school in Haifa. On the way home Ruthie, Hanna and I decided to stop for a cup of tea before the two-hour trip to Jerusalem. We had a choice of two routes back to the interchange. Our choice was normally to follow the coast south for about an hour, then to turn east to drive up to Jerusalem in the hill country. As we turned towards Jerusalem we realized that the traffic was very heavy. Later we discovered that half an hour before we came along and turned east a car bomb had exploded. It happened just about where we would have been if we had come earlier and had taken the other route. So our stop for a "cuppa" meant we missed the blast. We praised God for his protective hand on us.

As visitors to a country it is not what *we* do that counts. We move on – we are not going to be there all the time. It's what the local people do that is going to make the long-term difference. This underlies all my work – training is crucial.

34

"Retirement" – and more of the same

When I joined TLM my contract was until I reached sixty years, but it did not mean I was out immediately on my 60th birthday in 1989. By that time it was obvious that I had a unique role to play. I was travelling around Asia regularly visiting at least ten countries, teaching, doing surgery, consulting and encouraging people to improve the quality of their work for leprosy patients. A number of TLM people had continued working beyond their official retirement date. The mission was quite prepared to let me stay on but there was some concern about precedents.

So an unwritten arrangement was reached. Instead of my visiting card reading 'Adviser for Leprosy and Reconstruction Surgery for The Leprosy Mission in Asia', the word "Previously .... " was added – and I would continue as before! Whenever invited to teach or do surgery, I would go if possible and TLM would still pick up the expenses. In this way I would officially retire, collect my superannuation, and live in Sydney but be available on request.

A full calendar kept me working into 1989, although some trips took on a different aspect. At the Chittagong Medical School in Bangladesh I was presented with an award thanking me for the ten or more years that I'd been lecturing in that medical school. In Taiwan a similar thing happened in Taipei. The Minister for Health presented me with a large framed citation, a medal and a "thank you", as did the Taiwan Leprosy Relief Association – thank you for coming, thank you for helping. At a TLM conference in Nepal towards the end of the year I was officially farewelled as a full-time worker.

Back in Australia there were all sorts of matters to attend to. The mission had added extra money to my superannuation because I never really took my annual holiday, and rarely needed sick leave. My superannuation gives me a useful monthly allowance. My brother Bill and I thought it would be a good idea for me to settle in one of the attractive Anglican retirement villages around Sydney as he and his wife Gwen had done. Kathleen Collett also in due course moved into one, where she too has been able to continue her Christian ministry, hobbies and many other interests. We looked at several of them – Bill said I would need a shoehorn to fit into one unit. We decided it was a lost cause. There was no possible way that I could get all the equipment, the books, the teaching materials which I had accumulated over the previous forty years into one of these villas. Hopefully I would be able to sort things out and move into a retirement village later.

Obviously the best thing was to stay in Chatswood in the family home which was left to me when my mother died. Very conveniently my niece Ruth, a school principal, was able to move in too. She provided company and it was far better for the house to be occupied when I was away. In the nineties, until she moved out to a place of her own, Ruth and I had a Bible study group in our lounge on Sunday afternoon, sharing the leadership. It was excellent too to be more regularly part of my local church, where I could sing in the choir and occasionally play the organ. As a nomad, I knew all about the Church worldwide but had rarely been able to put roots down at home.

In 1990 and in most years after that I was able to attend the New South Wales Summer School of the Church Missionary Society at Katoomba in the Blue Mountains. It was always well worthwhile, bringing strong Bible teaching and encouraging awareness of current needs, and great opportunities to renew old acquaintances. It was one of the many special Christian gatherings I had had to forgo in the past.

For years I had planned to do many things that I never had time for while constantly travelling. In small snatches I had enjoyed sewing, embroidery, stamp collecting, gardening, cooking, photography – but there was so much more I wanted to do. There was rather a large garden to consider. Would I find time for them? Hah! A year after my supposed retirement my brother remarked, "You're not retired, you're re-treaded! It's the same you underneath."

In practice my "retirement" just meant new approaches to work – and lots more travelling. In 1991, as in 1982, I took the car ferry to Tasmania so I could drive myself around the island, attending TLM meetings and a medical conference. In 1992 I drove all the way north to Rockhampton, then went by bus to Townsville and back, taking TLM meetings en route, showing my slides and talking about the work we were doing in Christ's name to help the unwanted and disabled – especially, but not only, those with leprosy.

Those Australian journeys were arranged to fit in around overseas trips, as described under the headings of the various countries. But I must mention a couple of special trips. In 1991 I had made the last of my visits to the refugee camps on the Thai side of the Cambodian border. Dismantling was in progress and refugees were either migrating elsewhere under UN auspices, or returning home. We were concerned about the leprosy patients, so it was good to learn that the German organization *Malteser Hilfsdienst* would continue leprosy care in Cambodia.

I made a special trip to Anandaban in Nepal in 1992 to share in teaching five surgeons from China, who came to observe and learn about the reconstructive work. It was part of their extended tour to a number of different countries, sponsored by TLM, to assist in upgrading the rehabilitation programs in China.

The following year I visited Anandaban again, this time to coincide with a visit by Diana, Princess of Wales. She visited the leprosy hospital and spent about an hour walking around, talking to staff and patients, and sitting on the patients' beds. She was interested in the smallest details, and can be seen in one photo looking with interest at a makeshift traction that Dr Des Soares had constructed to treat an elderly patient's broken leg. A large plastic bottle of water served as the weight. Well, it worked! I was able to talk with her about the surgical rehabilitation program.

I was barely able to make that trip, as I had had a car accident two weeks before leaving. I suffered a compression fracture of my back, and wore a spinal brace throughout the trip. A grateful patient presented me with a handsome knobbly walking stick, but airport security viewed it with disfavour and it had to go in the hold. I still have it, though I did not really need it then or now – but one never knows!

It was a joy to me to be more involved in the hand surgeons' societies in various countries. I had demonstrated and taught some hand operations on visits home in the 1960s and 70s. Now I was asked to take a more active role, attending their conferences and clinics and teaching operations and techniques.

In the 1970s I had met Bruce Conolly while on furlough in Australia. He had recently returned to Australia from overseas studies and was taking up a teaching position in hand surgery. In the late 1970s he came to Thailand to work with me at Chiang Mai and taught me a lot of tricks and techniques. Ever after he was very happy to help whenever he could, and, when I was in Australia, he would ask me to see patients or attend meetings and give talks on what I was doing. By the time I retired he was the Associate Professor in Hand Surgery of two medical schools in Sydney, and is still keen to involve me wherever he feels my particular experience will help determine the best treatment for a patient or to teach trainees. Through him I was recognized as a consultant at one of the main hand clinics in Sydney. There are many people who know me only as a hand surgeon and are surprised when they realize that I have other irons in the fire – that I operate on hands, feet ***and*** faces!

Since 1990 there have been a number of Hand Surgery

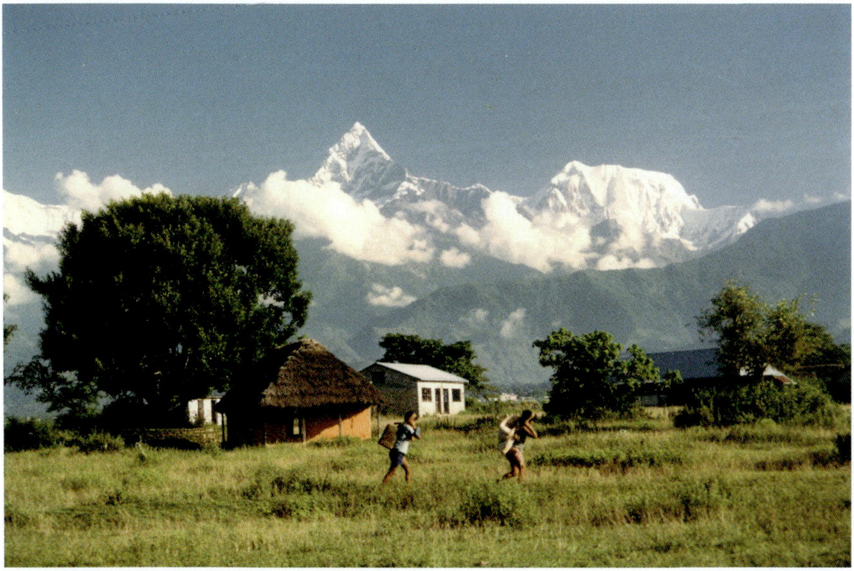

Green Pastures Hospital - Pokhara, Nepal

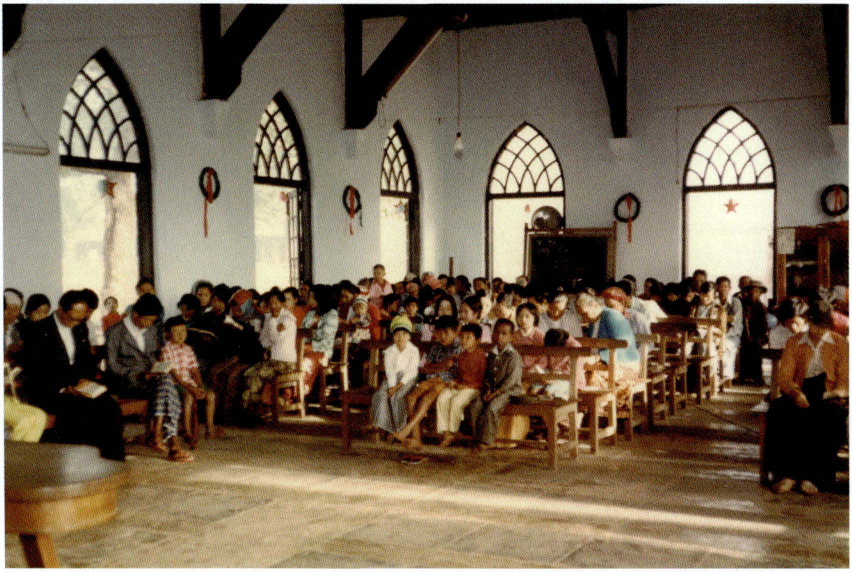

New Year's Day at old church at Moulmein Hospital - Burma

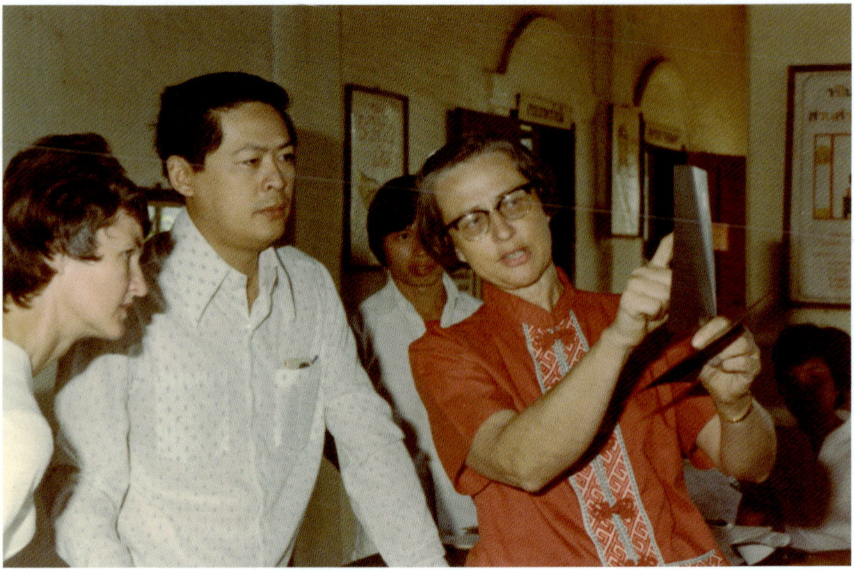

Grace Warren - teacher, Chiang Mai, Thailand, about 1978

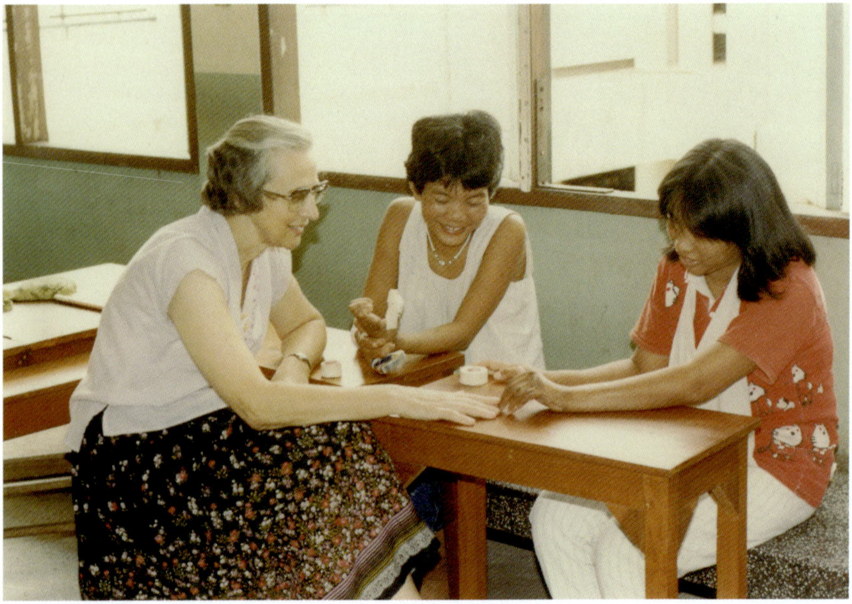

Dr Grace checks hand exercises at Manorom

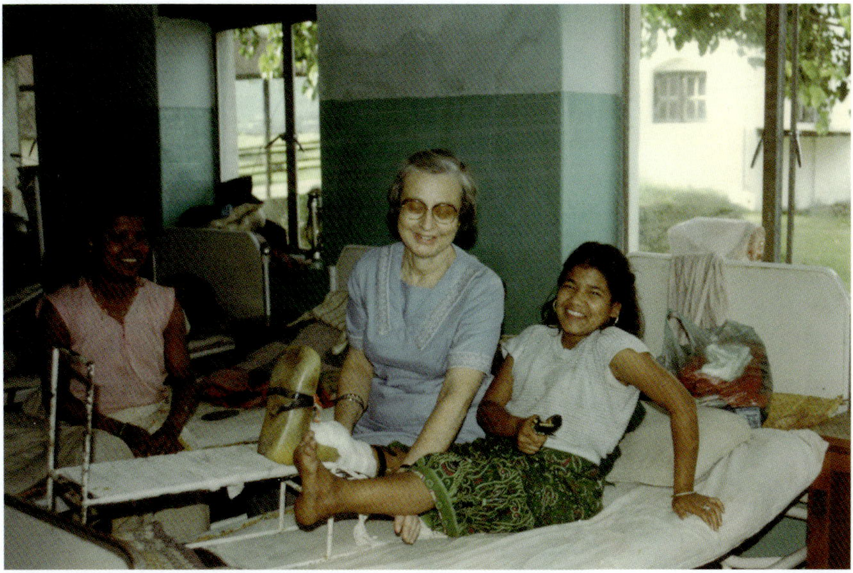

Post operative check after foot drop surgery - Pokhara, Nepal

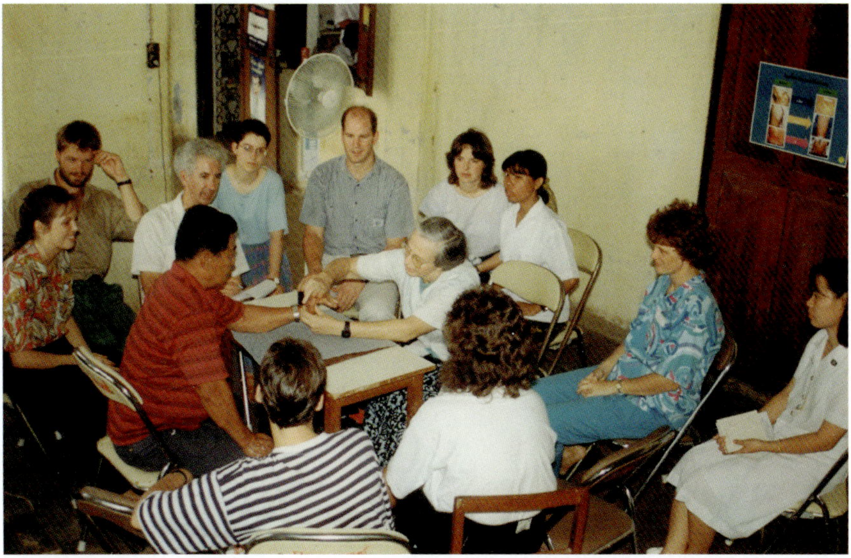

Teaching clinic in Chiang Mai, Thailand: Dr Trevor Smith (white shirt) & Dr Grace, observed by Dr Scott Murray – OMF (centre) and other staff and students

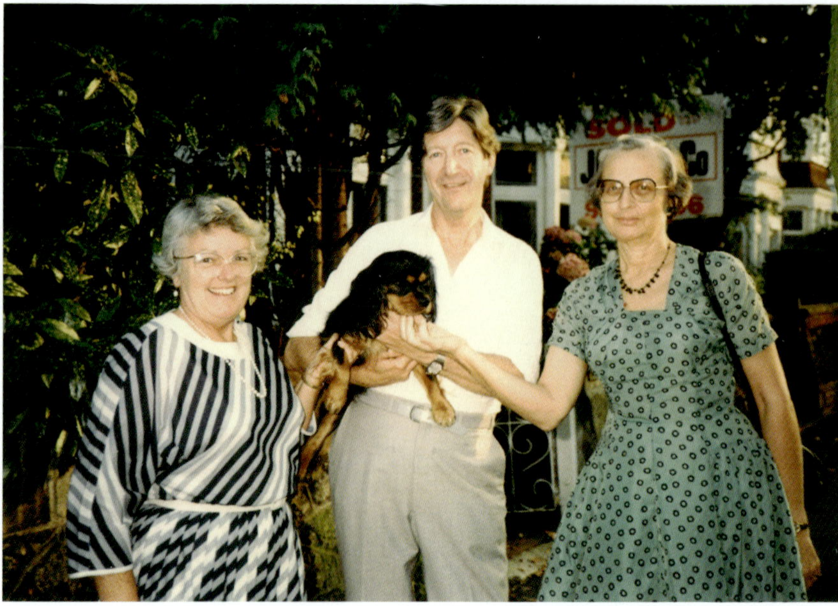

With TLM International Director Eddie, & Barbara Askew - England 1973

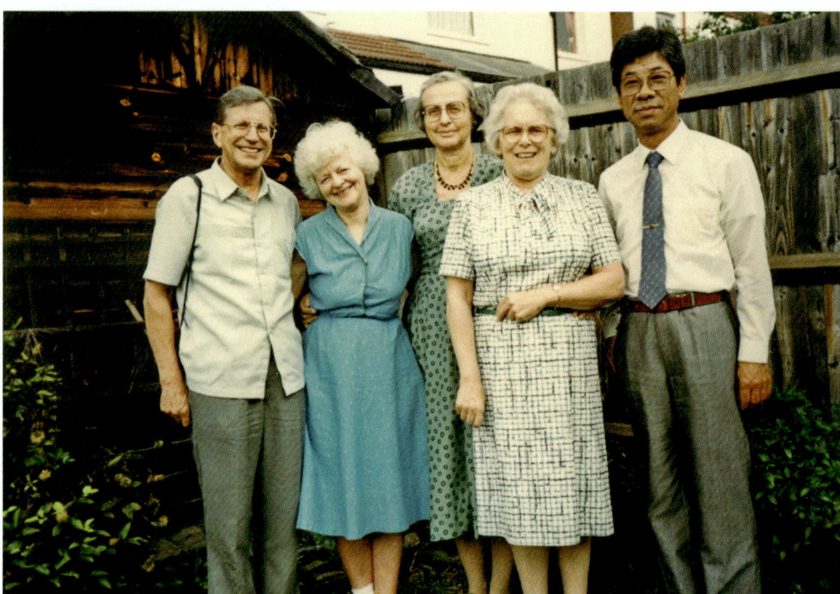

London reunion, 1973: Alan & Rena Waudby (Hay Ling Chau), Grace, Grace Bennett (Taegu hospital, South Korea), Mr Cho (Taegu administrator)

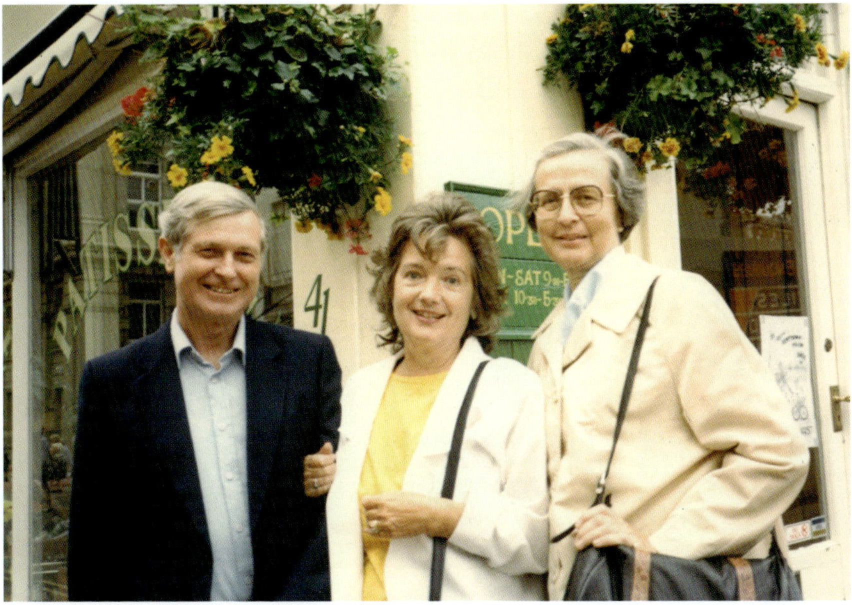

Dr Michael Waters & Mrs Valerie Waters with Grace - London 1973

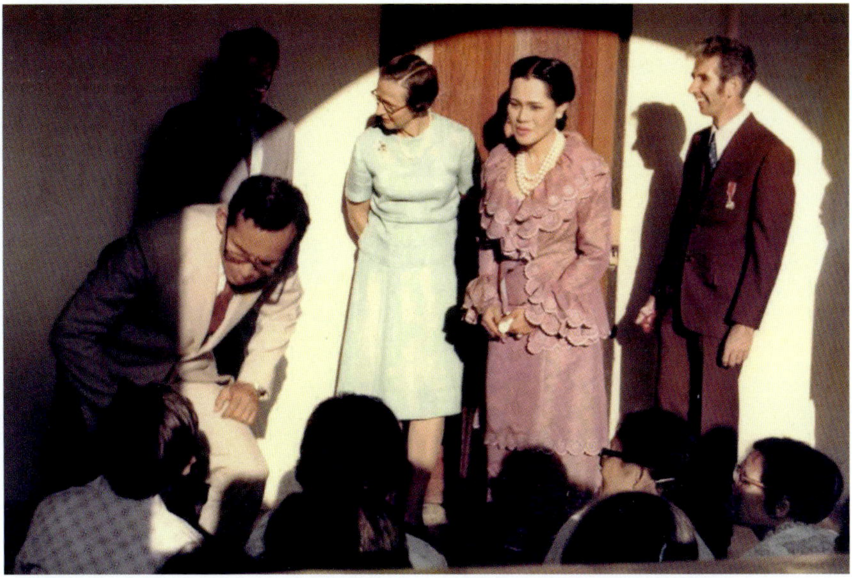

"The King & I" – H.M. The King of Thailand, Rev Richard Bryant, Dr Grace, H.M. Queen Sirikit, Dr Trevor Smith - 1977

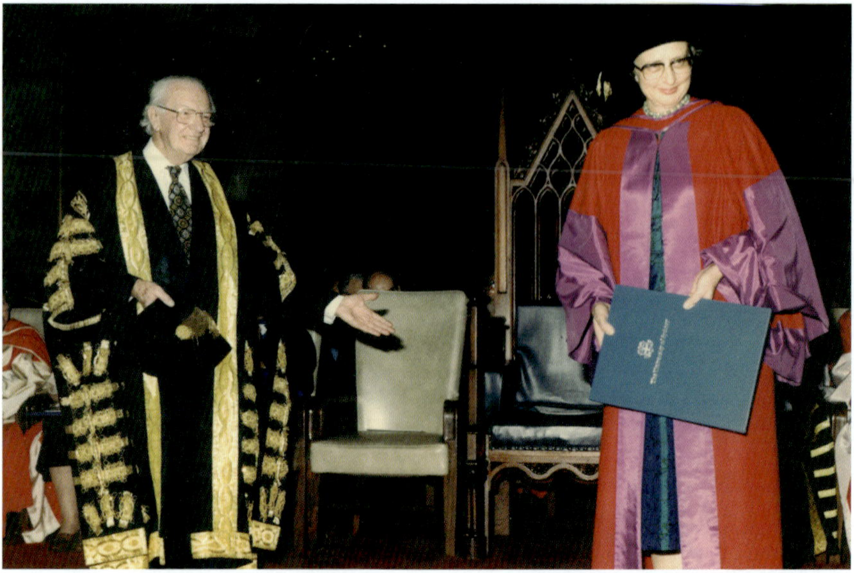

Grace receives MD, Honoris Causa, as Sydney University celebrates the centenary of women graduates - May 1985

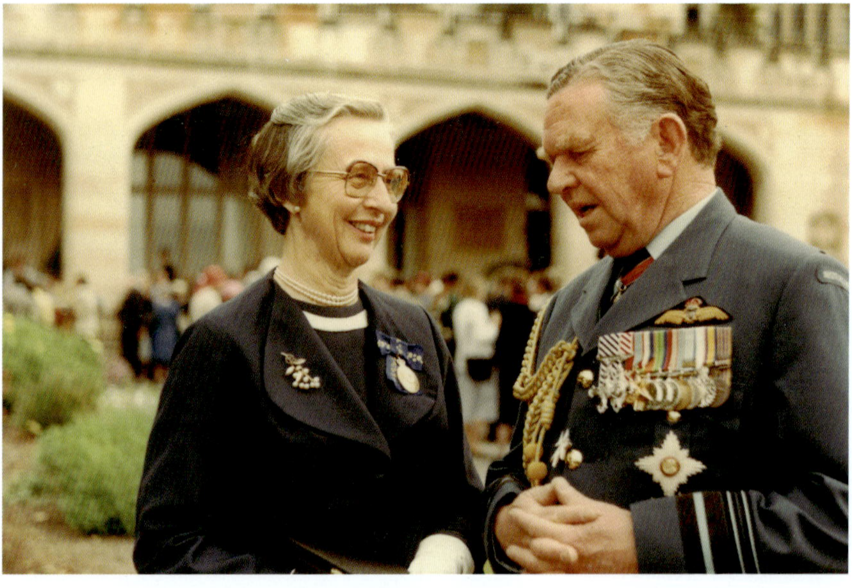

Chatting with the Governor of NSW Air Marshall Sir James Rowland upon presentation of A.M.- 1986

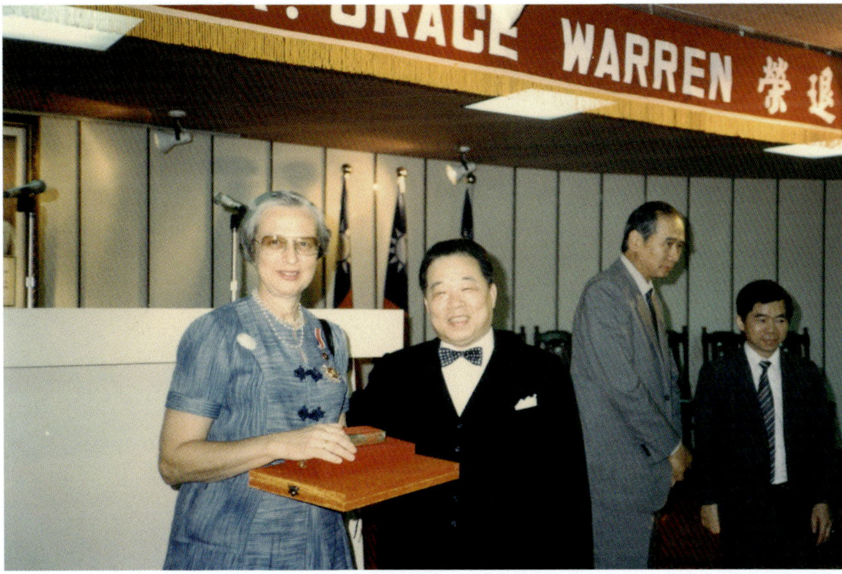

Grace Warren receives the Taiwan Health Department's Medal of Honour for 28 years of leprosy work in Taiwan - 13th May 1998

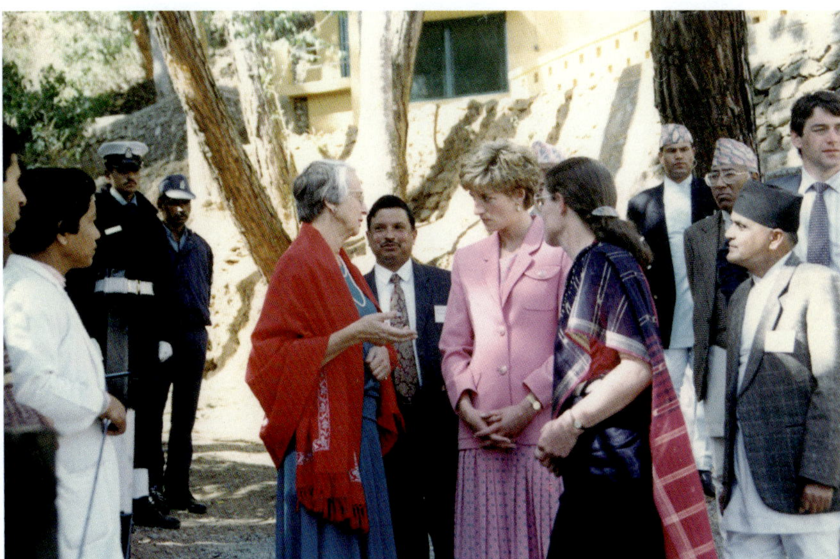

Grace talks to Princess Diana, Dr Ruth Butlin, Mr Pradeep Failbus (administrator) and other staff - Anandaban, Nepal 1993

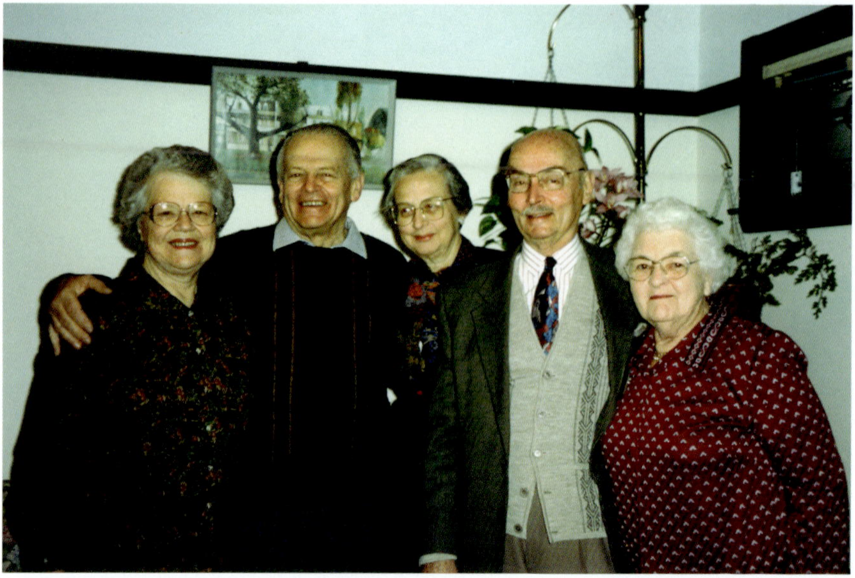

Warren family members - Sydney 2000: Ruth & David, Grace, Bill and Gwen

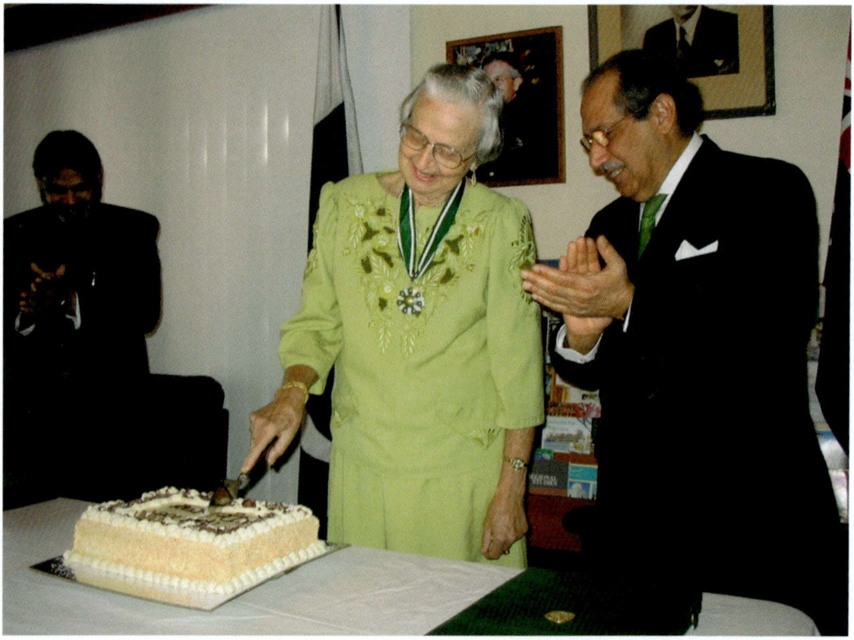

Grace receives the Star of Pakistan from the High Commissioner of Pakistan, H.E. Babar W Malik - 23rd March 2006

conferences at which I have been an invited speaker, such as presenting three technical "How to ... " papers – on tendon transfers – in Thailand. In 2005, I was a special guest at the Pakistan Hand Surgeons' conference at which I presented three papers and did one demonstration operation. Hand surgery is a most satisfying specialty. Usually one can see good results within a few months, and there is not the need for many months or even years of care nor the plaster casting often needed for the problem feet I deal with so much of the time.

I have operated on very few faces in Australia, but a couple of the Melbourne surgeons were very interested to learn my techniques to enable paralysed eyelids to shut again. Improved appearance can be obvious within six weeks – much quicker than with many other techniques.

In 1997 I was invited to speak at a fairly prestigious conference on the diabetic foot in Melbourne. Amongst the other speakers was Dr Andrew Bolton from UK, who then invited me to go to Great Malvern (UK) in May 1998 to speak at their biannual Diabetes Conference. This enabled me to share some of my experience with specialists from round the world and to rub shoulders with leaders in this specialty. It also led to writing a chapter to be included in the third edition of Professor Bolton's book on diabetes.

I again joined Professor Bolton in 1999 as a speaker at a diabetes conference in Jerusalem. That Israel trip was highlighted by lectures in several of their medical schools and working in the Military Hospital in Gaza. Next stop on that 1999 trip was Britain again, with more lectures for medical colleges, the Hospital for Tropical Diseases and TLM.

After 1993 I spent less time overseas, but travelled much more within Australia; to Perth in 1995, to speak at TLM meetings and to surgeons; to Cairns in 1996 to an orthopaedic conference, to present a paper on diabetic ulcers, and, on another occasion, to teach the local staff about the care of neuropathic feet, as so many diabetic patients amongst the indigenous population were needing care; and to Darwin, speaking at a medical conference, followed by a series of visits to work with surgeons, mainly on neuropathic feet.

In Australia's north a number of leprosy patients had foot problems, but by far the greater number of problem feet were due to diabetes. In Darwin, I was able to restart the foot care program, and demonstrate some of the operations that would help save the deformed feet that were the result of patients' (and doctors') failure to understand and apply proper care. Leprosy is still endemic in Northern Australia even though WHO states there are relatively few cases. So it is essential that medical personnel learn how to deal with the problems that leprosy patients encounter. Knowing good leprosy foot care will also improve the care for diabetics.

Life seemed to be settling into a more reasonable routine of travelling and teaching in Australia and overseas, when I was asked if I would visit the CIOMAL leprosy program in Phnom Penh, Cambodia, to assess and advise on their program, especially the rehabilitation services. Cambodia's leprosy program was devastated during the terrible Pol Pot years of civil war. The re-established government arranged for a Roman Catholic group, the Knights of the Order of Malta, to take responsibility for the program. Known by the acronym CIOMAL, they had set up a central referral and treatment centre for the management of complications and disabilities, and assisted in clinics. At one stage, a French doctor had been in charge, but he had left and CIOMAL was looking for a replacement. Some warned against OMF and TLM people because they wanted to convert people to Christianity. However CIOMAL could not find anyone who knew the disease and was willing to work with leprosy patients in such a difficult and neglected situation. Then they heard that Dr Steve Griffiths had come to Phnom Penh. He had the twin "disadvantages" of being an OMF worker and as having worked previously for The Leprosy Mission! But no-one could have been better equipped for the task.

Steve took on the challenge and as part of his efforts asked me to come over. In March 2002 on my first visit to Phnom Penh, I assessed facilities and ran a lecture course for the local doctors. But none of those who came to the course were prepared to take on leprosy full time. I spent time teaching the physiotherapists how to examine and record the patients' deformities, and to teach the patients the exercises that they needed to learn (and to **do**) before any surgery could be contemplated. There was no way we could correct the deformities of every leprosy patient in Cambodia, so we had to select the patients most willing to work hard at rehabilitation to produce good results.

An operation room had been built in the small hospital complex, but it was not in running order in 2002. We were able to use the facilities of the French (Roman Catholic) Hospital together with their staff to do surgery. On that visit we did foot-drop correction for seven patients. For each patient I worked with a local Khmer surgeon, hoping some would continue to do the procedures, but I am afraid they all had too many other priorities. I had to leave full instructions with the physiotherapists regarding rehabilitation. Fortunately, Steve knew the routine, and I was told that all the patients in the small hospital were out in the courtyard cheering on those who had had tendon transfers on the first day that they came outside to walk a decent distance. Their good results stimulated others to work on preparing their hands and feet for surgery.

Later that year Scott Murray, from OMF Manorom, went in to assess the operation room. CIOMAL had sought to set it up earlier, but the French doctor wanted it equipped like a French hospital and asked for a very expensive operating room light. The price tag made it unrealistic so plans did not get much further. However, Steve managed to get the US forces to fly in a used light from the USA as a gift. Although the glass got cracked en route, that did not alter its effectiveness. So we saved thousands of dollars that could be more usefully spent on other things. Scott then started going into Phnom Penh regularly and used the operation room to perform some reconstructive procedures.

When I went in to Cambodia again in February 2003, the new facilities were in use and we were able to do all our work in the CIOMAL compound. Next to the CIOMAL block is the ROSE block, where reconstruction surgery was being done for non-leprosy patients from all over Cambodia. Their surgeons often came to scrub in with us or to watch what we were doing, and I went across to that block sometimes to discuss their patients.

For several years I returned to Cambodia about every six months. By 2004 three surgeons, Scott Murray, Geoff Bird (another Aussie) and I were taking it in turns to shuttle in and out, getting on with surgery. However, in later 2005, it became more difficult to find those really ready to have surgery. Many patients would love to be able to say, "Oh yes, please operate and fix my hand or my foot, but do not ask **me** to do anything!" Those who were passive and unmotivated we did not want – I would only operate on those I knew would cooperate and work in their own rehabilitation. Also those who did come needed more attention in order to prepare them and teach them after surgery, overloading the staff. Outpatients with early deformity needed more attention, because giving them extra care could avert the need for surgery. So now we have reduced the number of surgical sessions annually. As Scott lives just over the border in Thailand, he now does most of the surgery and Geoff and I go less often.

But we are all open to changes in order to maintain a reasonable program of reconstructive surgery. In many centres, the numbers of patients asking for surgery reach a peak a few years after the program starts, after which the numbers fall off.

On trips to Cambodia I usually call in also to Thailand to help where I can. On one of these trips I was honoured with a ceremony held at Phrapradaeng (Bangkok Leprosy Hospital) to present me with a plaque in recognition of my many years of service in the leprosy program in Thailand.

35

Leprosy in Australia

After I retired I was asked to visit regularly the leprosy patients being treated at the Fairfield Infectious Diseases Hospital in Melbourne. As long ago as the seventies I had seen patients there occasionally. After some negotiations I agreed to become a consultant. I would go from Sydney to Melbourne as required and would receive a fee for service; I was not an employee of the hospital. That got me involved in caring for the ulcerated feet of some of their patients. There did not seem to be anyone else around Melbourne experienced in treating anaesthetic feet and prepared to give the time to look after them.

I also collected the job of advising on the ordinary medical treatment of patients with leprosy in Victoria and New South Wales. Many Australians are surprised to learn that there is any leprosy in Australia: in fact there are somewhere between two and three thousand cases. This was the number when there was a cumulative register, the register of every patient in Australia who had ever had leprosy and who was believed to be still alive. There were perhaps forty or fifty in Melbourne and a similar number in Sydney, scattered through the cities and suburbs. No one really knew exactly how many. The changes in the World Health Organization definition have resulted in official figures much lower than they should be for people who have leprosy or have had it.

Most Australian clinicians have never seen active leprosy and so one cannot expect them to recognise an early case, especially if the patient cannot or does not give a good history. One Asian, from a highly endemic country, who had been in Australia for a number of years, had spent three years, before I eventually saw him, going from one physician to another, then to dermatologists, because he had "funny" rings on his skin. To me the leprosy diagnosis was obvious. Instead of being dismayed, he was delighted to have a definite diagnosis, and more so when I could rustle up enough Cantonese to make myself understood without having to get an interpreter for every visit. He then brought his wife and daughter to be checked and has been very strict in attendance and is doing very well. However, those three lost years, without treatment, mean that there will be some otherwise preventable loss of sensation in his right hand.

A difficult case in the early 90s was a teenager from country NSW who had come as a refugee from a country where leprosy was certainly endemic. He appeared to be healthy when he arrived, but in his early teens he had gone to his local GP with something wrong with his foot, though the partial paralysis was not typical of leprosy. He was referred to one of the big teaching hospitals in Sydney where there was a doctor who 'knew all about leprosy'. He prescribed anti-leprosy medication, and, when the foot did not get any better, gave him corticosteroids, which I have mentioned before. These did not help. The leg was getting more and more painful, with less and less movement.

Then the GP heard about me and asked if I could see him. Immediately I knew full well that this was **not** leprosy. In fact it proved to be a cancer. The reaction when we gave that verdict was completely unexpected. I have rarely seen parents so relieved. In their culture and social strata leprosy carried a terrible stigma. That was the last thing they would want one of their children to have. A cancer – well, anyone can get cancer. Fortunately I was able to contact someone at the teaching hospital in Sydney. I arranged for a biopsy of the nerve and it turned out to have been virtually destroyed by a malignancy.

Another surgeon operated to remove the cancer and surrounding tissues, which meant that the leg was paralysed below the knee. As a result the boy had a completely floppy foot and hated wearing the splint that the hospital had provided. I was then able to operate so that he ended up with a foot that was functional. He was able to run along the edge of the swimming pool with his friends without that unsightly calliper on his leg and without his foot flapping in the breeze. They got all the cancer out and it is not a worry now. He's now well into his twenties. He's married to a delightful girl from his own racial group and they have a child.

Yes, it is just one story, but I praise God that I was around and had the privilege first of saving this boy's life and then enabling him to function normally enough to enjoy his life. I am thankful that I know enough, first about leprosy – when it is and is not present – then about the necessary reconstructive surgery, to be able to help people like this.

Meanwhile, I had got involved with the problems of leprosy patients in Victoria. There was a woman who had had ulcers, ulcers, and more ulcers. Every time she got an ulcer she had a bit more of her foot chopped off. We were able to stop that, and although over the next ten to twelve years we could not completely stop the deterioration, we were able to keep her walking on her own two feet for nearly twenty years after her original problems commenced. Eventually she had to have one leg amputated, to improve her general health, but she was able to live alone and look after herself. She had her flat modified, and used a wheel chair.

Quite a lot of the work that I do with leprosy patients now is handled by phone, email or other electronic means. In this way I can tell them how to fix some of their problems. Others I have to arrange to visit. In the 1990s and on into the new century, in between overseas trips, I am going regularly to Melbourne to see patients and do surgery. I also visit a number of other centres scattered over Australia.

From about the mid 1990s I was regularly visiting Prince Henry, the old Coast Hospital (Infectious Diseases) in Sydney, and later the new Prince of Wales Hospital, for consultation about leprosy patients. The variety of people with leprosy in Australia is fascinating. There are a few aboriginal patients who originally contracted the disease in the north. But most down south are immigrants or Australians who have contracted leprosy while living and working overseas.

Migrants often have interesting stories. One young man came into Australia on a student visa, intending to qualify and then obtain a permanent visa. He had been in Australia for some months when a skin lesion showed up on his lower rib cage. A retired Chinese doctor saw it and knew very well what it was. The boy's GP had called it psoriasis, just one of the many skin conditions that leprosy resembles. When we questioned him about it, we found the patient knew he had had the lesion the whole time but he begged us PLEASE not to tell his parents that he had leprosy. The other problem was that, if we let him go back to his Asian country for his summer holidays, he would not be allowed back into Australia, because active leprosy was not welcome in immigration. We managed to arrange for his treatment and he was able to gain permanent residency.

There was another Asian teenager in Adelaide who was seen by a neurologist with a nerve lesion on his left hand. The fingers on his left hand would not straighten and he could not use them properly. The neurologist had a pretty good idea as to what the diagnosis was, but, as he had not had much to do with leprosy, he felt that it would be a bit presumptuous to state it. It so happened that I was going to Adelaide to speak at some TLM meetings, and the mission had arranged for me to stay with this neurologist, who said, "I hope you do not mind, but I've arranged for you to speak at a neurology breakfast on Monday morning. There is a boy with an ulnar deformity and I would like you to examine him in front of the neurologists and show them how you examine nerves." He told me where the boy had come from and how long he had been in the country.

There must have been twenty or thirty of the specialists, trainees and medical students at this breakfast and I was introduced. They brought the boy in – a nice looking young fellow, about 15 years old. When he raised his left hand the ring finger and the little finger were very obviously bent – classically so. It was what we call an ulnar nerve paralysis – a very common leprosy ailment. I carefully examined both hands and demonstrated the difference between the two hands, one paralysed and one not. Then I proceeded to feel the rest of the nerves on his arms and found that virtually every nerve was larger and harder than normal. I could show those neurologists these abnormal nerves, some of them visible, but most able to be palpated or felt, which few of those watching would ever have encountered before. They might merely have read of them in a textbook. They were vying with each other to come and feel!

There were nerves on his neck and forehead; on his legs were more large nerves even though he did not have muscle weakness. So I then asked him if he had ever had anything wrong with his skin. "No," he said. "No patches?" "No," he said. "Let's have a look," I said. There on his lower chest was a perfect ring, red, a bit thickened and raised. "Oh," I said "that is interesting. What's that?" "Nothing" he said. I looked elsewhere and found a few more patches, not as obvious. So I looked at the neurologist with a big grin. I knew what he was thinking. We may have seemed heartless to be jubilant at a firm leprosy diagnosis, but in reality it was good news for this boy. There was good hope for his future.

We reconstructed the story. With all the wars in S.E. Asia the boy's family had been displaced from their land. As a six year old he had wandered around, eking out a living. Then the family secured a boat passage and lived in refugee camps. He had lost his parents at some stage, so that he was now an orphan. The Red Cross had eventually brought him from a camp in Singapore to an adopting family in Adelaide. Now in his early teens he was being loved and looked after and properly fed. His general health had improved markedly. His other medical problems and minor infections were dealt with. He was no longer anaemic. Previously he was such a sick little boy, it was probably all that his body could do to keep him alive, with all the acute illnesses that could have killed him. But the leprosy infection was lurking. That first ring on his chest could have appeared when he was six or seven years old. They are usually just one of the signs of the type of leprosy that will heal itself. But then came the privation, the escape, the boats, the refugee camps, losing his parents. It's all stress, with the result that his disease was no longer adequately controlled. Without his showing obvious signs of leprosy during those years, the bacteria were spreading widely in the nerves throughout his body.

Eventually, when he was generally healthier, his own T-lymphocytes, the white cells whose job it is to attack bacteria, started working against the leprosy baccilli in the nerves, causing swelling. This swelling cut the blood supply in some nerves and he developed paralysis of the ulnar muscles of his left hand. The neurologist asked how to treat him. I prescribed the full anti-leprosy medication as well as steroids in his case because we wanted to save those nerves if at all possible. Three months later the neurologist phoned me. The boy had just been in to see him. "That hand has now recovered. His nerves are all settling down extremely well – and the trainees, the students, are looking for nerves everywhere now. They had never seen half of those nerves before."

That morning's work not only helped one young fellow to regain a useful hand and to forget the fears of leprosy, but helped all of the trainees so that in future they will be much better able to examine patients with nerve problems. Very few people would have realised what was wrong. God has ways of using people like me both to help individuals in great need and to convey necessary teaching to others, in order to enhance and multiply our service.

I heard a story from a nurse who had worked overseas in leprosy for years and was now working back in Australia in an emergency department. One evening a woman came in with some strange lesions on her arms. The doctor in charge was puzzled. The nurse said, "Those are leprosy lesions are not they?" He looked horrified. He would never have thought of leprosy. She was right, and, as it happened, the patient knew full well that she had leprosy but was not going to tell anyone. So the doctor asked for that nurse to work with him in the clinics where they had lots of migrants presenting with all sorts of illnesses which were not always easily diagnosed – including, at times, leprosy. So this is one of the problems – supporting staff as well as doctors have had very little experience in leprosy and do not always know what to look for. There are not many with experience like that nurse.

At Fairfield Hospital, Melbourne, one day I was asked to see a Chinese gentleman of nearly 70, Ah So, who had been living in Australia for fifteen years. He had had leprosy that had left him with bilateral foot-drop. He had fairly recently remarried and had a small son, two or three years of age. The doctor who referred him to me said "Can you do anything for his feet so that he can walk more easily?" and I said, "Sure!" I did the foot correction with one of the local surgeons. A physiotherapist, Barbara, then took over and taught him how to use the muscle which I had transferred so that he could lift his toes off the ground and walk better: first surgery for one foot and then for the other. Barbara loved doing that sort of physiotherapy for my patients. Many of her patients were chronic cases needing daily physio for survival and to keep them as mobile as possible, but as Barbara said "Your patients, I know that within three months they will be off and out and I won't have to worry about them again. They're so rewarding!"

Ah So learned to use the second muscle properly and to walk quite well. He could even kick a football around with his young son – a whole new lease of life!

36

CMT – "Shark's Marine Teeth"

One day in 1993 I was asked to see a young woman whose feet were quite deformed and was told that she had *Charcot Marie Tooth* syndrome. The name comes from the three surgeons, two French and one British, who first described this inherited abnormality of the nervous system. By the way, I love the story of one patient who informed her doctor that she had "shark's marine teeth"!

Usually abbreviated as CMT, the condition causes abnormal muscle function with a slowly progressive loss of muscle power particularly in the feet. It can also affect the hands, and in severe cases, other parts of the body. It is one of the familial neuropathies written about in Chapter 30. People with CMT also have altered sensation in their feet so that, though they may not feel true pain, they describe uncomfortable sensations in their feet as pain. I go to great lengths to teach my trainees and students that they must differentiate between this neuropathic "pain" due to nerves not functioning normally and the normal pain caused by, an infection or a fracture. Because their feet are not normal in shape, and because they do not feel normal pain, such patients sometimes develop ulcers on their feet very similar to those of leprosy or diabetic patients.

Here was another group of patients who needed special care very similar to what we had developed for our leprosy patients – and another group who would benefit eventually from my book on the care of neuropathic limbs. A patient, Jean, was sent to me; could I do anything for her feet? In 1993 I knew very little about CMT, but I looked at her feet, as I would look at any leprosy patient's foot, and said, "Well, I think we can. I cannot guarantee it, but there are surgical procedures which we can do that will help to give a better shape and more stable walking."

I found an orthopaedic surgeon who was interested in working with me, and we admitted her to a private hospital on Sydney's North Shore. We operated there on the first foot, put her into walking plaster soon after surgery, and kept her in it for nine months – the duration my leprosy patients needed. Nobody that I knew of had done this sort of surgery for CMT before, and many people said that it would not be effective. I was confident however, because of my success with leprosy patients. When the first plaster came off Jean was so thrilled with the shape of her foot and her ability to walk that she begged me to go ahead and do the second foot, please. Well, that was the beginning of a flood.

While teaching Jean to walk again we arranged for the podiatrist at the Concord Hospital, where I had been doing the Diabetic Clinic to teach her to care for her feet and also to modify an inner sole in her shoe to give increased stability, so she could wear a basically normal shoe. Jean could buy these at a much better price than the special orthopaedic boots that she had previously worn.

A couple of months after I had done the second of Jean's feet another CMT patient, Susan, rang up and asked could she see me. Professor Nicholson, who was doing the genetic studies at Concord Hospital, had recommended that she should have her ankles arthrodesed – that is, stiffened or fused. The paralysis in Susan's feet caused her constantly to go over on her ankles. But her podiatrist, when she heard, said, "I do not think arthrodesis should be necessary. You go and see Dr Grace Warren."

I arranged for Susan to come to Professor Nade's clinic. She produced Professor Nicholson's letter saying that she had CMT, and recommending arthrodesis. Professor Nade and I examined her muscles and checked her X-rays. He said to me, "I think that if you do your usual tendon transfers, that will solve the problem." So we got her onto his operating list. Before the surgery a rather irate Professor Nicholson phoned me, demanding to know why I was interfering. "She has been sent to have her ankle arthrodesed, and that is what she needs," he said. It was just as well that I had taken her to Syd Nade, because I was able to say, "Well, the Professor of Orthopaedics at Westmead Hospital says that she does not need arthrodesis of her ankle."

As a professor of neurology, Professor Nicholson knew about her nerve problems and muscle weakness and that genetically she had CMT. But he acknowledged that he did not really know what else surgeons could do to help her ankle problem. All he wanted was for her to have stable ankles. Three months after my surgery Susan walked into his office at Concord Hospital and said, "Look at me now! I can wear sandals again that I haven't been able to wear for years! My foot is stable. It is pain free and I do not have to wear special shoes any more." From then on Professor Nicholson started sending CMT patients to me – a continuous line of them through 1997 and 1998 and continuing up till now in 2006.

In 2001 I was working with Dr Andrew Ellis, orthopaedic surgeon and senior lecturer at Sydney's Royal North Shore Hospital, doing some of these tendon transfers with him. He was very keen to learn because he realized that he could use these techniques to deal with other problems. Dr Ellis was involved also in the orthopaedic work of the army. Whenever the army was posted overseas they were prepared to do what they could to meet the surgical needs of the local people. He could see that the tendon work that I was doing could be very useful to him when he was dealing with patients with deformities after trauma or war wounds.

Operating together on these patients Andrew and I got it down to a fine art. If such a patient needs surgery, they usually need both feet operated on, though maybe one is not as bad as the other. CMT however is a progressive disease, and, even if one muscle works this year, it may not work next year. Part of the art is to look ahead and do as much as possible in one operation. I also learned to assess the progress of the disease, and we developed a technique whereby we were able to rebalance the foot in one operation so that hopefully no further surgery would be needed – and by working together we could do both feet at once! Many people, who had operated on CMT using tendon work in the past, were confronted with the fact that patients required repeated operations time after time as further deformities developed, because the surgeon had only corrected the present problem.

Because Professor Nicholson has sent me so many of these patients, I am now able to predict that if the peroneal muscle has gone now, the next muscle to be paralyzed will be the anterior one, followed by the one to the toes. Eventually only two foot muscles will really be functioning. The two at the heel which are the ones used when you want to stand on your toes or when you turn your heel in. So by moving one of them, the *tibialis posterior*, to the front of the foot just as we do in leprosy, we can leave the patient with a balanced movement of the ankle. It will go up and down when the patient is walking, enabling what looks to be a near normal gait in normal shoes.

Andrew was very involved in teaching, and he decided that what we were doing had never really been written up in the medical journals and that it ought to be. So, at the end of 2001, I was extremely busy collecting data, the records of the various patients that I had operated on since that first patient in 1994. Andrew's research assistant, Eileen, was able to draw up a big table on the computer with all the information and the material. Andrew appointed one of the trainees, Sindy Vrancic who is hoping eventually to be an orthopaedic surgeon, to review all our results and present them first at an orthopaedic meeting and then at a general surgical meeting. In 2002 Andrew presented a research paper written in theory by the four of us, which included the results of 43 of these reconstructed feet on which I had worked. As far as I know there is no other series anywhere near as big as ours of tendon transfers for the reconstruction of CMT feet.

In the year 2002 I operated on maybe another ten to fourteen feet of patients with CMT and on a number of other patients with similar problems. Some of them are not suitable for this type of surgery; for some we have devised another operation which will help them. Where possible I now refer them to one of my trainee surgeons who has been working with me, and who can now do this same procedure. If the surgeon wants me to, I will still go and work with him so that if anything unusual crops up during the surgery we can discuss it together and do what is best for the patient.

So from 1996 I have seen a constant growth in the number of surgeons using these modifications of Dr Brand's original techniques. As a result there are so many delighted patients – patients who claim that the tendon transfers have made the world of difference to their quality of life.

I was asked to see 12 year old Sally in her last year of primary school. Her feet were twisting quite badly because of CMT. She was having problems running though she still did manage to run, and her mother too had had very serious problems. So the family was not looking forward to the fact that Sally's feet would probably become more and more deformed as she grew older. We operated on her in early December, as soon as she had finished her final primary school exams. So she was in plaster for Christmas. Then in January she was back in hospital to have the plaster casts removed and to be taught how to walk using the transferred tendons in her feet. When school resumed in early February she was to commence high school. Sally was able to enrol at her new school with feet that appeared normal, walking with a normal gait. Six months after surgery when we were reviewing her, she came in grinning and said, "I am now playing soccer in my new school!" That was a triumph for us because there was no way that Sally could have played soccer before. We were able to give her back the ability to take part in normal activities, even sport, with her peers at school. We could not guarantee that her feet would not get worse later, but we expected that they would remain in functional shape and position with no need for major surgery. About five years later she did require some modifications, but it was so satisfying being able to do that for a teenager.

After we had reconstructed the feet of Alan, another teenager, he won silver medals in table tennis in the Disabled Games. He could never play before because he kept tripping over his feet. With his tendons relocated however, he no longer had the problem of clumsiness. He was able to walk quite well – and he swam extremely well and won races in the interschool swimming championships, not just the Disabled Games. It's a tremendous thrill to be able to give back to these young people the possibility of a normal or near-normal life. One of the things I am praying for is that more people will realize the potential of the tendon transfers that Paul Brand used to such good effect amongst the leprosy patients of Asia, and that we have been able to bring to people needing the same sort of care here in Australia.

Another fascinating set of patients came to me as a result of a television program back in 1984. Dr Leigh Delbridge was then a lecturer in endocrinology surgery; he later became Professor of Surgery at Royal North Shore Hospital. Leigh and I were working one morning on the foot of a patient who had diabetes, when a camera crew arrived from the ABC – the Australian Broadcasting Corporation. They had pre-arranged to film what we were doing and to record some statements about the conservative type of surgery that I was doing for patients with abnormal pain perception.

They shaped this into an excellent program shown on television Australia-wide one Friday evening.

After that television program three people had rung up the ABC, each individually, until they found out who I was and where they could get in touch with me. They were distantly related but had never met before; they met for the first time in a waiting room of Professor Thomas Reeve at the Royal North Shore Hospital. Each of them required a different management. That was the beginning of my association with a group of genetically impaired patients that is known in Australian medical literature as 'The Edmunds family'.

All were descendants of one immigrant who came to Australia in about 1800 and married a Mr Edmunds. They had a large family and their offspring mostly had good sized families. The original woman however carried a gene for an abnormality of nerve function. A large proportion of her descendants had feet and/or hands which either did not feel pain normally or in which the muscles became weak and were paralysed. In males this problem usually started to appear in their teens, and in the women not until they were over twenty. My experience with such people over the following twenty years indicated many variations. They are a fascinating group of patients to work with: patients who have some feeling in their hands and feet, but not what we would class as normal. They could have odd sensations of pins and needles, aches and pains in their feet, yet they could walk on sharp objects and not feel it as pain, with a result that many of them developed ulcers very similar to those in diabetic or leprosy patients.

Eventually I treated about forty 'cousins' – people from the same extended family – with these problems. I am still warmly welcomed into many of their homes as if I were family myself, because I and my colleagues have been able to make such a difference to their lives and outlook. Some members were facing amputations. I did not think they needed an amputation. One woman who had been told that she needed both feet off, is still walking round on those feet twenty years later. She has had problems with them certainly, but they are still her feet, in relatively good condition and serving her well!

So together with CMT patients, the Edmunds family form part of the story of my official "retirement" here in Australia. In the past five years I have had still more referrals for many other patients with many variations of the same problems – partial paralysis and deformity and altered pain perception. To help them has been tremendously rewarding for me, and the patients are usually so grateful, especially those who have been told: "Nothing can be done," or "We cannot cure you – you just have to learn to live with it." It's true that we cannot *cure* many of them, but we can help make their lives significantly better. That is one of the joys for me in being a surgeon.

37

Westmead Hospital and Neuropathy

In the 1990s I attended clinics at Sydney's Westmead Hospital once or twice a week. People who had diabetes or some similar foot problem connected with nerve damage were being referred to me. Working with Professor Sydney Nade, Dr James McGrath and Dr James Wong, I started "collecting feet". I also had to teach nurses how to look after them. I began using plaster casts. The word soon got round that we were saving feet that other people said could not be saved.

I was also asked, early in 1990, to give a lecture to a group of podiatrists specializing in treating diabetic feet. In 1984 I had met the "Edmunds family", with their neuropathic foot problems. One member of the family had lived in Newcastle: I had put a cast on his foot and achieved the healing of an ulcer which had been there for years. A very complimentary letter came from Newcastle podiatrist, Mr Alan Boyes, on how effective my cast was in obtaining healing of this ulcer, which Alan had been seeing intermittently for many years. He was one of a group of podiatrists who did a lot of work for patients with diabetes, and who invited me to give a lecture to podiatrists one night at the Ryde Hospital.

I turned up with my usual material on how to look after the neuropathic foot, put on casts and treat ulcers. At the end one of the senior podiatrists came up and said, "That was fascinating, Dr Warren. You say 'Do this'; other people say 'Try this' ". I guess that is part of my experience. I know what is going to work, and the patients soon know that, if they want me to help them to deal with their feet which may be partly paralysed and have impaired sensation, they have to do their part.

I am well aware that many podiatrists do not agree with what I recommend. Repeatedly, they say that diabetic patients should not care for their own feet, they should go to a proper podiatrist. More easily said than done! There are not enough podiatrists in Sydney to deal with all the diabetic feet that should really be checked on a daily basis, and even fewer podiatrists outside of Sydney. The only thing is for the patients themselves to be able to look after their feet every day, or to have a carer to do it for them, and visit a podiatrist if they can to check it is being done correctly.

As a result of that lecture, some podiatrists got me involved in advising about their patients' feet; so I was going to the Concord Hospital Diabetic Clinic fairly frequently to see some of them and discuss treatment. That led to involvement with Professor Garth Nicholson, a neurologist very interested in genetic studies and in the problems of patients who have been born with abnormal sensation. So I was appointed as a consultant in his department at Concord Hospital. Some of the diabetic patients from Concord Hospital who required surgery, I took over to Westmead to operate on with Professor Nade.

It was at Westmead in 2000 that I saw Daren, whose story I began to tell in Chapter 1. When I took him on, the first thing I did was to make him a plaster cast – a special one – so that we could take it off at regular intervals, check the ulcer, dress it and then replace the cast. But he was able to walk in it. With his instability and his previous nerve and muscle damage, he could not have walked without using that left leg at all, such as by walking on the right leg with a pair of crutches. And so we fitted him with a removable total contact cast until the wound had improved enough for surgery.

Three months later Daren had that surgery and went into a new cast made to accommodate the changed shape of his foot. As healing proceeded, the cast was changed several times, and, after six months, the foot was healed. The ulcer had healed and the remaining bones were in much better shape. Now he was able to start learning to walk again without the plaster cast. A long process, but by the following Christmas, he was able to stay out of that cast all day. He still needs to take good care of that foot, and both his feet will always require extra care, because his original spinal injury means that the loss of pain perception is permanent. He has to rely on his eyes and hands to take care of his feet and to prevent more ulcers and problems. The following January he came back to my clinic. As he walked in I commented, "Why are you wearing the cast? I said you could leave that off now unless there are problems." He grinned, presented me with a huge bunch of flowers, and said, "Well, I am working in the Fire Brigade stores at present, and when I have the cast on, the men help me by carrying their own supplies – so I do not have to use the foot so much! But when I am home, or when I go visiting or driving the car, I have it out of the cast."

Wise man! He had learned full well what so many patients never learn – that a foot like his, nerve damaged and lacking full pain sensation, is very vulnerable. He has to guard it with great care. As one of my other patients with a similar problem said, "I realize that I have a finite number of steps ahead of me – when they are used up the leg will need to come off or it will have worn away. It depends on me!"

In the 1990s I spent a lot of time travelling, making connections, trying to contact surgeons and other clinicians who were prepared to learn what I had found to be useful and to put it into practice. There is now a small network of surgeons in Australia who are doing the same sort of tendon transfers and foot reconstruction by bone surgery that I have been doing. I hope that they will be able to continue to do them for many years to come. Then more people like Daren could keep feet otherwise likely to be amputated.

Mark was another one who had been told very emphatically that his foot had to come off. Well, it was not just his foot: he was told his circulation was so bad he would have to lose his leg above the knee! At this stage of the game I was asked to see him. Again came the plaster cast.

The tissues were then protected from rubbing and knocks and were able to heal themselves. The foot showed improvement, but it was later obvious that some infected bone would have to be removed. Again at surgery we removed only the dead tissues and reshaped what was left. Instead of losing his whole leg, Mark probably lost only about one quarter of his foot. He was very pleased and went into one of my special casts. With his foot healing nicely, he could look forward to getting a new pair of regular shoes with a special insert to compensate for what was removed. Using this insert, he has had no problems for over four years.

Our bodies have a remarkable ability to heal. It is absolutely fascinating when one works with Mother Nature – or more accurately, with God, the ultimate Healer. It is only in this present generation that people expect things to heal yesterday, and are not prepared to allow the time necessary for wounds to heal themselves. So Mark was grateful and amazed that we could save three quarters of his own foot. The surgeon who worked with me was intrigued, not having seen this sort of approach before. For Mark a few more weeks in a cast was worth it to keep his foot – and in any case he could still walk around in the cast.

One of the most satisfying things for me is that I have found a number of younger surgeons prepared to learn what I was doing and to apply it to their work. The principles that we learnt doing leprosy work in third world countries, where we had to work with minimal equipment at minimal expense, and in the face of a horror of amputation and its great social stigma, has changed the whole outlook. The result is that many feet can be saved **if** the patient is prepared to work with me. And I put that **IF** in very big letters because many patients will come with problems of various types expecting me to work magic: to fix their foot in one operation so that they do not have to do anything or ever have to worry about it again.

It does not work like that because feet like these will need continued care for many, many months or years. To keep a foot and keep it useful, that is the price to be paid; if not, there are plenty of doctors who will chop it off and order an artificial leg. With my conservative work, I can always take further action at a later date. Even if amputation has to happen eventually, at least the patient knows that we did all we could to try to save that limb.

In 1999 I got a thrill. I received a letter informing me that I had been nominated to receive an inaugural award in honour of Sir Edward Hughes, the past president of the Australasian College of Surgeons who had died in the previous year. This award was to be given to somebody with real ability in surgery, who had done a lot to help others. I was to share that award with John Hargrave. I have mentioned John elsewhere (Chapter 19) – an Australian who qualified a year or two after I did and then worked as a Government Medical Officer in the Northern Territory in the 1970s and 80s, doing significant leprosy work among indigenous people. He was also involved in research surgery with people from Sydney University and did reconstructive surgery. Like me, John had never done formal surgical training. I had taught him some of his first reconstructive surgery in Hong Kong in about 1965.

John and I received that award together at a dinner one night in Tasmania, where John lived quietly in retirement. TLM wanted me to do some deputation there and it made sense to organize for it to be at approximately the same time as the award so that John did not have to travel interstate. Of course I've retired too – supposedly – but I am afraid I do not live quietly anywhere!

38

Getting the Word Out

Although I would much rather wield a scalpel than a pen (or a computer), I have done lots of writing over the years. I wrote notes for my students about leprosy in 1960, and then later about surgical techniques and the surgery I did, and I was often asked when all this would be published. Well, I did not really know, but in 1990 I realized that I needed a computer – and I did not know the first thing about them. This was obviously something I had to learn. It was rather expensive. A portable one, a laptop, cost about A$5,000 in those days – far more than I could spare. I happened to mention this to one of my friends at church, and he enquired of a friend of his who was with IBM.

The outcome was that Professor Tom Reeve, from the Royal North Shore Hospital, arranged a celebration in his rooms. At this the local IBM representative gave me a cheque for A$5,000 to buy myself a portable computer to use for recording my surgical procedures and copying materials to pass on to others. That was an absolute windfall. And IBM was generous enough to say that I did not need to buy one of theirs! The IBM man had to admit later that, at that time, they had nothing as small and light as my little Toshiba. That little computer worked very hard; in 1990-1991 I slaved away trying to get the written notes from my work over the previous twenty years into some sort of order so that they could be published as a book.

I never was a literary person. At school I was told that my writing and spelling were atrocious, and my written English was certainly never good. Writing articles was really hard work for me – much more writing a whole book! But I collected quite a pile of material, and the next step was to find who would publish it for a completely unknown author. I sent out summaries of the forthcoming book, showing its style, content and illustrations, to various medical publishers.

Professor Bruce Conolly helpfully recommended a firm who had published for him, but negotiations dragged on for several years. At the last minute the editor said "No, we won't do it because we are not sure who will buy it. It's not for surgeons, it is not for physicians, it is not for podiatrists. We do not know where to list it." The problem was that a practical manual covering all aspects of caring for the neuropathic foot just did not fit anywhere, although as far as we could tell such a book had never been published before.

I happened to mention the sadly lapsed project when I was in London, where I was seeing patients at the Hospital for Tropical Diseases. Frank Tovey, who had worked in leprosy in South India in the 1960s, was now involved in diabetic foot work in England, having had helped develop a suitable shoe for diabetic patients to protect their feet and reduce the incidence of ulceration. Frank suggested Parthenon Publishers as he knew the manager. The manager was dubious at first, but, as Frank Tovey had requested it, he eventually agreed to take it on – if I was sure we would be able to sell at least one printing.

Despite my lack of gifts in these directions, praise God that he has the answers. I had known for years that God wanted me to write a book on neuropathy – that it was an important part of my work as a whole. One day at Westmead Hospital I had mentioned my attempts to Professor Sydney Nade, Professor of Orthopaedics at Sydney University, and he had offered to help me. Having written several books himself he was an excellent teacher, and appreciated what I was doing to help those with neuropathic feet and he knew what others needed to know. He went through my drafts and edited them, adding and subtracting material. Hence, by the time I sent it to Parthenon it was already reorganized into a reasonable order, trimmed and corrected, saving their editor a great deal of time. Syd knew what was necessary to get the message through. So I was extremely grateful to him for helping to get that book off the ground. It is doubtful if I could have found anyone better able to help if I had gone hunting worldwide.

So in 1997-98, letters, faxes, computer floppies and piles of paper flew back and forth between Australia and England, eventually followed by the proofs, the corrections and illustrations – a huge volume of work. All the book's photographs were mine, from patients I had dealt with, both in Asia and in Australia. Line drawings were done for me by Ron Dawes, who became the mission's NSW State Secretary during the time that I was preparing the book. All this took vast amounts of time, yet there were many delays because I was getting more and more requests to go all over Australia, teaching the very aspects of care that are covered in the book.

Eventually the book was published in July 1999. The manager of Parthenon agreed to a print run of 2000 hard-backs. Then TLM ordered 500 at a special pre-publication price to give to leprosy hospitals worldwide. That was very satisfying to me, because the mission had initially stated that the book was not needed. However, I have been assured time and time again, and still recently, that it has unique value as the only book that deals with the subject of neuropathy as an entity and not just as a complication of some other disease.

Moreover it is a practical manual – it tells the reader what they can do and what they can teach the patient to do to look after themselves. It's written in my usual down-to-earth plain style that is not full of big technical medical terms. This is one of the things I have been criticized about – that when I am lecturing I do not use enough impressive medical or technical terminology. But it is not necessary. Dr Stanley Browne, whom I greatly admire, once said that if you know what you're talking about you can use one syllable words that everybody can understand. That is partly what I've done.

TLM Australia ordered and paid for a further 1000 laminated copies more suitable for tropical places, and Parthenon gave them to us a very special price. That now enables us to offer them to third world countries below the original cost price. I am now wondering if more might be needed!

In the early sixties I began a circular letter which became known as *Warren's Wanderings*. It was originally sent just to family and close friends, but later to supporters and interested colleagues around the world. Over 500 copies were posted each issue. These were the people who provided the most essential support of all by praying for our work. Stanley Browne, in his book *Leprosy – New hope and continuing challenge* (first published by TLM in 1966), accented the need of prayer when he quoted the words of the founder of the mission, Wellesley Bailey. "The Leprosy Mission was 'cradled in prayer' and its greatest need today is the continuing believing prayer of God's people. The vast and ever-growing task undertaken by the mission must be activated by prayer if it is to accomplish eternal as well as temporal good"; and "the work is always in need of dedicated men and women, Christian first, foremost and throughout, who will devote their skills and their knowledge, in the name of Jesus Christ, to those who suffer from leprosy. The task does not lessen, despite the gratifying dimensions of the successes already registered in the campaign against leprosy." (Ch 10 P82, 1977 ed.)

After my official retirement, some thought I would have plenty of time to prepare and give lectures and write articles and notes. They do not realize how long it takes me to prepare lectures. Initially I illustrated them with my 35mm Kodachrome slides. It was relatively easy to reshuffle a set, changing it to suit the needs of the audience, so I rarely gave the same lecture twice. Now most groups asking for lectures require Power Point presentations, prepared by computer. These take me much longer to prepare: it takes me a long time to scan photos to transfer to the computer. The first long – 45 minute – lecture I gave using Power Point took me about 400 hours' work – but I did manage to do it myself! After that learning exercise, preparing talks did not take me so long, but it is still more time-consuming now than in the past.

I have literally thousands of separate teaching slides, as well as slide sets, and many of them are used in articles that I have published. In the last few years I have had the assistance of Ron Dawes, who does excellent black and white drawings as illustrations. I have written special book chapters and articles on aspects of neuropathy. Ron and I have also worked together to produce a two-part article on the care of diabetic feet for general practitioners, which has been reproduced by other publications. Articles in major medical magazines and journals are widely distributed and reach many readers. So you can see that God has opened up many ways of getting the message of "*rest and protect*" out to the clinicians who care for those in danger of destroying their feet – and to diabetics and others who are themselves at risk.

Early in 1990 I went to Melbourne by train in order to consult about patients in Melbourne hospitals, and to be a speaker at the Christian Medical and Dental Fellowship (CMDF) Conference held at Lorne on the southern coast of Victoria. I was advised against the long drive by car, but that meant that I had to borrow or hire a vehicle in Melbourne. Before long I was driving myself for most of my trips. That certainly meant that I saw a lot more of Australia than I would have otherwise. To have my own car was certainly more convenient for carrying my projector, teaching materials and surgical instruments and so on. I soon had places along the main highway between Sydney and Melbourne where I could stay with friends or patients. From that time up to the present I have been to Melbourne for a few days or weeks about every three months, often being able to arrange trips to fit in with meetings, TLM deputation or other events.

Accompanying me on those interstate trips was the new Toshiba computer. (But now I am on my third computer.) About 2002 I borrowed a dictaphone from the Leprosy Mission office and commenced recording this story. I guess it is obvious that I am a person who hates wasting time! It occurred to me that I could usefully occupy those hours spent driving – and have an activity to keep me awake too. So I talked as I drove, recording what I could recall of many fascinating events of my life, my work and my travels. I filled tape after tape, and these were eventually transcribed verbatim onto computer disks by willing, long-suffering friends, members of my own local church, St Paul's Anglican Church, Chatswood. I am most grateful to first, Judy Hodges and later Gwen Compton, who between them did that transcribing work; without them this book would never have come into being. Then Lesley Hicks, also a St Paul's member, an experienced writer and an author in her own right, in close consultation with me, took on the daunting task of shaping this rather rough, complicated and enormously long oral account into the much shortened written form you are now reading. All have worked unpaid.

That 1990 CMDF meeting was the first of a series in which I took part. Previously I had not been in Australia for many of their meetings. My career was so unusual and so obviously showed the touch of God's hand, that I was several times asked to share my experiences with the younger doctors and trainees, who were seeking to know what they could do as Christian doctors who desired to follow God's leading.

It is most encouraging to see the numbers of young doctors and other medical professionals willing, even in this materialistic age, to "go anywhere" in obedience to Christ's call to preach the gospel **and** to heal the sick as part of his ongoing work in the world. Missions like CMS and OMF – the two, besides TLM itself, with which I have had most to do – are seeing increasing numbers of well-qualified short-term volunteers, who in many cases go on to become long term workers.

39

Into the Future

In these last two years, 2005/6, there have been far fewer trips and meetings, giving me more time to work on this book and to start setting my house in order ready to move into a retirement place. I have so much stuff that needs to be disposed of, and it is far from easy to find the right place for things that I know can be of real use to the right person.

But life is never all work. One bright spot this year was to meet up again with Daren who dubbed me "Doctor Number 49". Daren is still working in the Fire Brigade, with responsibility for some of the training, and he is very happy with his feet. Granted they will never be completely normal, being neuropathic, they give him little trouble – no more ulcers, and he can wear normal shoes. He was glad and so were we, that he did not need to consult Doctor Number 50!

About the time we met him earlier this year (2006), I also received information that I was to receive the Sitara-i-Pakistan – The Star of Pakistan – at a special ceremony at the Pakistan High Commission in Canberra on 23rd March, Pakistan's National Day. The Star is one of Pakistan's top civilian awards, equivalent to the AM in Australia or the MBE in the UK. It was given in my case for Humanitarian Service in Reconstructive Surgery for under-privileged people in Pakistan. I had commenced that work in 1967 and had been teaching others to do it ever since – a period of almost 40 years.

It was a lovely day – members of my family and some friends came to join me as we gathered with some of Canberra's Pakistani community. After the raising of the flag and Islamic prayers, we went indoors where the citation was read and His Excellency Mr

Babar W. Malik, High Commissioner for Pakistan in Australia, presented the medal before quite a crowd. I made a short speech and cut a special cake. Refreshments followed in the garden. A very special occasion indeed. My main regret was that I had not been able to receive the award in Pakistan, where the pleasure could have been shared with those who had worked with me through all the years.

That day and that award – one of many – enabled me to stop and think of all the ways my Lord has led me and how he has fulfilled his promises in so many situations. As a teenager, of course, I had no idea where God would lead me. I knew I wanted to serve him but I had no high ambitions to get to the top of any tree. I was always in the middle in achievement and expected to stay that way. Yet my life and my career have worked out in ways far more rewarding than any I could possibly have imagined.

God apparently gave me an ability to improvise and make-do, "thinking outside the square" to find the best solution to a problem. I guess it is also a variation of the engineering and inventive ability that runs in the family. For example, rebalancing tendon function is really mainly a matter of ropes and pulleys. My father was an engineer and a handyman and reshaping feet is really carpentry, another skill in which I had been encouraged early in life!

At present it seems right that I should continue a certain amount of travelling, teaching and lecturing. I do not run a regular surgical practice in Australia these days, but I am allowed to teach others and this suits me admirably. Whenever someone comes to me who requires surgery I refer them to somebody – a younger surgeon – who wants to learn how to do the operation that I think is the right one, and we work together. This is not just for that patient's benefit but also for the benefit of those who will consult that surgeon in future.

The gifts God gives are ours to share with others. Now I can say there are literally hundreds, if not thousands, of people around the world who are accepted in their communities and are able to support themselves or their families because God caused their paths to cross with mine. Yes, I have received recognition and honours; but I want to thank countless friends and supporters, and above all, to give to God all the glory and praise.

What does the future hold? Who knows? One of Eddie Askew's verses seems to express it better than I can.

Lord,
you are the way.
Not simply final destination
but journey too.
And as I travel on
I sense your presence.
Your life in mine, my life in yours, dovetailed and intimate.
And when I cannot see the way ahead
With all the clarity I'd like,
Give me the grace to trust.
That is the hardest part at times,
But, Lord, if you trust me
Then surely I am right
To put my trust in you. *

* Eddie Askew, Encounters, TLM Int., 2004, page 123

Index

Note: Due to space restrictions, this index is neither fully comprehensive nor exhaustive. It covers mainly medical information and people's names, but generally excludes geographical place names.